"This book is a wonderful tool fc companion. As suggested in the book, I also found in my veterinary practice that what was being fed was the most important factor in the health outcome. Improving the diet, as suggested here, will often restore health without need of any other treatment. Don't tell my colleagues, but if you follow this plan you will have far fewer veterinary bills."

—*Richard H. Pitcairn, D.V.M., Ph.D., co-author of*
Dr. Pitcairn's Complete Guide to Natural Health
for Dogs & Cats

"Jan Allegretti's Fresh & Flexible meal plan is so much like my recommendations for feeding my clients' animal families that I almost can't separate the two! For almost 40 years I've watched my clients' animals improve their health with just fresh-food diet changes, and it's clear that fresh, wholesome, varied food is optimum for all animals and people alike. Jump in, don't be afraid, use Jan's guidelines and watch the beauty and magic begin!"

—*Dee Blanco, D.V.M., C.V.H., C.V.A., Santa Fe,*
New Mexico

"Groundbreaking, thought provoking, and visionary. The Fresh & Flexible Meal Plan is THE nutritional resource that guardians have eagerly been waiting for.

"Drawing on decades of experience, Allegretti demystifies the preparation of fresh, home-cooked meals for our animal friends, eliminating the confusion that often accompanies their nutrition. This book offers a powerful new solution that just may offer your beloved companion the one thing we all want for them and for us…time. When my dog was diagnosed with kidney cancer at age 14, feeding her the Fresh & Flexible way added years to her life, a gift that I believe not only benefited her longevity, but my happiness as well.

"Get ready to revolutionize the way you feed your companions and watch them thrive! If it works for my dogs, I suspect it will work for yours."

—*Carlyn Montes De Oca, author of* Dog as My Doctor, Cat as My Nurse and Paws for the Good Stuff

"A friend told me once that the best work is done by those having pure intentions. Jan Allegretti is one of the most purely-intentioned people I know. Instead of preferring a few species (including humans) over others, Allegretti breaks down the walls between our beloved cats and dogs and the beautiful and amazing cows, sheep, pigs, and fish that we typically feed them. Read this book if you are tired of closing your eyes to the labels on your dog and cat food. Follow these easy guidelines, and then relish in your companion's glowing health, even as you embrace your continued love for our wider world and all of its denizens."

—*Wendy Jensen, D.V.M., author of* Practical Handbook of Veterinary Homeopathy: Healing Our Companion Animals from the Inside Out

"Along with Dr. Todd Cooney, I was introduced to Jan Allegretti's Fresh & Flexible meal plan at our annual veterinary homeopathic meeting. As homeopaths, we know that inadequate diet can be a major obstacle to cure. We are also experiencing increased contamination and toxicity in our commercial food sources. Feeding like this is a conscious, mindful choice toward helping our animals reach better health. In addition, this method has significant beneficial environmental and ethical ramifications.

"What really resonated for me was the way connection and nurturing in the healing process was enhanced by providing fresh and quality food for our animal companions. I also loved how we could eat healthily together and not depend on questionable sources in commercial foods. It is empowering to control what is going into my dog's bowl.

"Along the way, my clients also began to see the results in their own animals. Many started by gradually adding whole food additions into their animal's present diet, starting the transition where they were able. Jan's presentation is straightforward, sensible, and simple, and it can be started right now."

—*Marybeth Minter, D.V.M., Mariposa Veterinary Service, Kenab, Utah*

"Many of my new patients who come in with years of chronic problems are on processed kibble. The caregivers think their little friends are getting old and slowing down. I tell them to change the diet to fresh-made, loving food. After a week of all fresh foods, they report back telling me they now have energy they never could have expected to see again in their furry friends.

"The problem is similar in human caregivers. Whole food helps to repair and regenerate because it is alive and packed with life energy. Processed food that is prepared over a 4- to 6-day period is overcooked and devoid of life energy—it is no longer viable.

"I have heard many times over from clients that their best friend feels so much better, is more mobile, and playing again with his or her toys just by changing to a nutritious diet! There can be no doubt that food is essential for well-being, undeniably."

—*Rosemary Manziano, D.V.M., C.V.H., C.V.C. Colts Neck Animal Clinic, Colts Neck, New Jersey*

"Jan Allegretti's *The Fresh & Flexible Meal Plan* is a valuable complement to the available guides for companion animal food preparation. Her emphasis on daily *variety* of the food groups is absolutely key to the success of this feeding method and is unique compared to standard recipe references. This book is for all styles of feeding, including vegan. Very few references are available for making balanced vegan diets, and the Fresh & Flexible method will assist your study and understanding of how to be successful. Here is an opportunity and outline for feeding a fresh, balanced diet that, when properly implemented, will promote overall wellness, and improve and support all other natural therapies provided."

—*Lisa Brienen, D.V.M., C.V.H.*
Holistic Veterinarian

THE FRESH & FLEXIBLE™ MEAL PLAN

Also by Jan Allegretti…

The Complete Holistic Dog Book:
Home Health Care for Our Canine Companions

Listen to the Silence:
Lessons from Trees and Other Masters

THE FRESH & FLEXIBLE™ MEAL PLAN

The Easiest, Most Nutritious Way to Feed Your Dog and Cat

JAN ALLEGRETTI, D.Vet.Hom.

Silent Voices Press

A Silent Voices Press Book
Silent Voices Press was created to advocate for
those whose voices are too often unheard.
Silent Voices Press, Ukiah, California, U.S.A.

Cover by Damonza

Interior formatting and design revisions by Mark Coleman
Mark@MarkColemanDesign.com

This book and the work of Holistic Animal Health and Advocacy are
supported by the Fred & Jean Allegretti Foundation

ISBN 979-8-9882814-0-5

For Tino

Contents

Foreword

by Lisa Melling, D.V.M., C.V.H., C.V.S.M.T.
Co-Founder, Faculty Instructor, Veterinary Homeopathy Institute

Veterinary schools and many post-graduate continuing education lectures place a high value on feeding companion animals a processed, commercial kibble because it is "nutritionally complete and balanced." There is a great deal of fear and even shame that feeding "table scraps" leads to digestive upset, allergies, pancreatitis, and obesity. Where has our common sense gone? How have dogs lived alongside us for over 17,000 years, and cats for more than half that time, sharing our diets in the centuries before commercial kibble became available, and still managed to thrive? Would any of us eat from the same bag of processed food at every meal simply because our doctor assured us it is perfectly balanced? Absolutely not.

When I was introduced to Jan's Fresh & Flexible plan at our annual veterinary homeopathy meeting, I was teaching my clients to feed home-cooked meals following recipes created by veterinary nutritionists, and supplemented to meet AAFCO standards. Jan's proposal that we could simply share our healthy meals with our animal companions stretched my mind to new levels. At first, I was very uneasy about letting go of structured recipes, and I told her so. With a sweet smile, Jan asked me if I follow recipes for every meal I eat, and answered all my other questions with intelligence and patience. I was hooked.

In the years since, I have been sharing my healthy plant-based meals with the animals in my life. I am grateful that the Fresh & Flexible plan gives me the option of feeding plant proteins, which supports my ethical beliefs that no animal should have to die so they can be eaten by me or my animal friends. I have come to recognize that dogs are "flexitarians"…they have adapted alongside us to share whatever diet we are eating—as long as it is varied, fresh, and healthy. While cats are not as flexible in their nutritional requirements, it only takes a little more knowledge, creativity, and careful supplementation to share our healthy meals with them as well.

In my veterinary practice, I recommend the Fresh & Flexible plan for my patients—to help heal those with chronic illness and keep the healthy ones strong and vital. In our efforts to educate more veterinarians in the art of creating healthy, fresh diets for their patients, Veterinary Homeopathy Institute has partnered with Jan to provide the nutritional training in our post-graduate homeopathy course. I am forever grateful to her for helping me and countless others become better healers and caregivers for our animal companions.

Introduction

by Todd Cooney, D.V.M., M.S., C.V.H.
Animal Wellness Center, Natural Animal Consulting[1]

Jan Allegretti offers a revolutionary but simple approach to feeding our furry friends—easy to follow, and certain to result in happier, healthier animals. Her approach to nutrition reminds me of another revolutionary thinker, Dr. Samuel Hahnemann, and his system of medicine developed in the late 18th / early 19th century, known as homeopathy. And similar to homeopathy, her method is criticized by some, but proven to work by any who dare to follow.

Jan fell in love with homeopathy in the 1980s, and is a longtime advocate for animal rights, welfare, and wellness. She began consulting work with an emphasis on nutrition and holistic animal care, and became a highly sought expert in these areas.

She is committed to enhancing awareness of our connection to all life on earth, and sharing her knowledge and experience with all who share a passion for the wellbeing of our animal friends.

I first learned of her Fresh & Flexible meal plan at an annual gathering of veterinary homeopaths in Arizona, hosted by Dr. Richard Pitcairn. She shared her feeding plan, and amazing results, showing pictures and videos of several older Great Danes. These rescue dogs lived almost twice the average life span for the breed, eating only the Fresh & Flexible diet using plant-based foods. Most of us marveled at this information, and its ramifications for our own lives and clinical work with dogs. That day I began to rethink my assumptions about animal nutrition.

Returning to busy veterinary practice life in Indiana, I shared the principles of Fresh & Flexible feeding with my clients, and also began to see the results in some of my animal patients. Caregivers appreciated this "no recipe" method of feeding, a refreshing alternative to the myriad books on canine and feline nutrition. The radical idea of sharing our food with our

---

[1]NaturalAnimalConsulting.com

animals opened many minds to a new level of shared compassion. I loved sharing this idea of saving ourselves and our animal companions by eating the same healthy foods, without the artificial classification of "human grade" and "animal grade" ingredients.

Several cases of stubborn "skin allergy" and "ear infections" are now back to normal after trying the Fresh & Flexible diet, as well as many "sensitive stomach" cases, and just plain finicky eaters. Many clients comment on the fact that they eat this way themselves, but never realized their companions could also. Just as it is a very liberating feeling to break away from the mainstream medical model, and use homeopathy for most treatments, it is also very freeing to be independent of commercial foods, and know exactly what we are feeding our animal friends.

My confidence in this method grew, as I followed the results in my patients and my own dogs. This book will serve as an invaluable guide to many, offering a liberating way of keeping your animals healthy and happy, while sharing this journey with our furry friends, and improving our own lives too.

May it be a blessing to many.

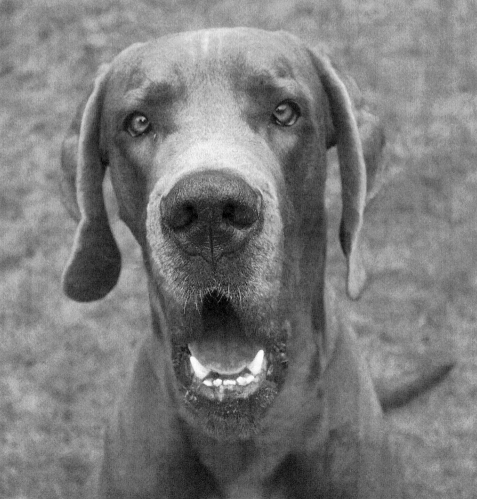

1 part one
The Search for the Most Nutritious Diet

part one

chapter 1

Why an Excellent Diet Is Essential for Good Health

In August 2007, I adopted a sweet, loving, 2½-year-old Great Dane. Initially I named her Tila, but in time I realized she exuded such a vibrant, beautiful presence that she needed more name than that, so she became Tila Marie. But it took a while for that vitality to emerge.

When I first brought Tila home, she was terribly underweight, even after gaining some twelve pounds while in foster care. Her spine, ribs, and hip bones were clearly visible under a coat that was dull and splotchy, with patches of brown mingled with the black. And she was sick. She had a respiratory infection and a severe yeast infection in her ears, and when she moved it seemed she didn't have quite enough strength to manage her tall, lanky body. While dealing with all of that, she had recently given birth.

I had traveled to Colorado to pick her up, and on the drive home to California I continued to feed her the high-end kibble and canned food her foster family had been giving her; I didn't want to make changes when we had a four-day trip ahead of us. It took a lot of coaxing to get her to eat each morning and evening in our hotel room, and I was concerned.

Tila's first meal in her new home was a bowl of lentils, brown rice, and broccoli, all of it cooked until it was nice and soft so it would be easy for her to digest, with a drizzle of flaxseed oil and a sprinkle of nutritional yeast on top. She barely gave it a sniff before diving in and licking her bowl clean. Then she turned to me with a look that was clearly asking for more. That was her introduction to the Fresh & Flexible meal plan.

In the weeks that followed, Tila ate a variety of fresh, whole foods, all prepared here in my kitchen, something different every day. There was an assortment of higher-protein foods, complex carbohydrates like quinoa or winter squash, and plenty of fresh fruits and vegetables. She seemed to enjoy the adventure of discovering what new flavors would appear in her bowl each day.

I have a photo of Tila on that August afternoon when we first met at a park in Denver, then another taken here on our rural hilltop in early March. The difference is striking. In less than seven months, her dull, splotchy, brownish-black coat had become a glossy blue-black that glistened in the sun, radiating health and vitality. Well-formed muscles cover her once-visible bones, and she stands tall and strong, ready to race across the meadow. The best part is the huge smile that parts those marvelous, droopy, Great Dane lips.

By the time I met Tila, I had been feeding the Fresh & Flexible meal plan here at home for several years, as well as writing about it and teaching it in workshops and to clients. It's a radical new way of feeding our dogs and cats using the same principles we use to feed ourselves—no kibble, canned, or packaged food, and no recipes to follow—just a varied diet of fresh, whole foods, straight from the kitchen. I knew it was what Tila needed, because I had seen again and again the power it has to benefit animals dealing with all kinds of health issues. Questions about food had become the place I began any consultation, because I already knew that an excellent diet is the key to achieving and maintaining good health—and that poor-quality food alone can be a cause of many of the problems that lead clients to reach out to me. I also knew that, when the diet is inadequate, the most well-chosen homeopathic remedy, herb, supplement, or even pharmaceutical is unlikely to restore the kind of vibrant good health that every dog and cat deserves, and that every loving caregiver seeks.

I'm trained as a veterinary homeopath, and have enormous appreciation for the ability of homeopathy to address a vast range of physical and emotional disturbances. I also know that herbs are an excellent way to gently restore balance and relieve discomfort. Most often, when a new client contacts me they expect a conversation about homeopathic remedies or herbs that might be helpful. It makes sense, because that's become the most common approach in our medical system: Find a pill that will fix the problem. I understand—and don't entirely disagree—and I'm happy to explore homeopathy, herbs, and supplements as possible solutions.

But for me, the place to start is with the diet. That's because I've learned over the years that if we fix the diet, many—*many*—problems go away.

That's right. If we improve the diet before we explore other therapies, often there's no need for any other therapy. In many cases the illness or discomfort goes away with no need for additional treatment. On the other hand, if the animal is treated with homeopathy, herbs, or, yes, pharmaceuticals, without first removing the cause of illness—such as an inappropriate diet—he may improve for a while, but once the medicine is withdrawn, the problem is likely to return.

> "If we fix the diet, many—*many*—problems go away."

It's clear, then, that an excellent diet is foundational to good health—even essential to achieving optimal health and longevity. Doctors of human medicine have begun to recognize how important this is for their patients, and many now prescribe dietary changes to address chronic illnesses like heart disease, diabetes, arthritis, obesity, and even cancer, and also to reduce the risk that a healthy patient will develop these illnesses. Their recommendations usually start with a varied diet of fresh, whole, minimally processed foods—much like what I recommend in the Fresh & Flexible meal plan. I've seen how this approach can help address those same illnesses in our nonhuman family members. It's my hope that it will become a first step toward health and healing for all our dogs and cats.

....

Finally, in case you're wondering…I had the great privilege of sharing my life with Tila Marie for 9½ years, and she ate the Fresh & Flexible way the whole time. She left this world one warm California day in January at the age of 12. I was fortunate to live with two other rescued Great Danes, Savannah and Tiffany, before and after Tila. Each of them came to me after a challenging start in life, and each had her own set of health issues when we met…and, like Tila Marie, Savannah and Tiffany enjoyed the Fresh & Flexible plan from the day they came home until they died, both at the age of 13, well past a Dane's "expected life span" of 8 to 10 years. I believe their excellent diet contributed to their long, healthy, and happy lives.

....

Please join me in exploring why changing the way we think about feeding our dogs and cats is so important. In the pages that follow, you'll find everything you need to make an informed choice, as well as a complete guide to how you can implement the Fresh & Flexible meal plan in your own kitchen, for your own best friend. You'll even discover how easy (really!) it can be.

Let's get started.

chapter 2

Commercial Food Is Not the Answer

We've been sharing our caves, tents, and homes with dogs and cats for tens of thousands of years, but packaged foods as we know them today have only been around since the 1950s. In that short amount of time, processed foods have become the go-to way to feed our nonhuman family members. They first gained popularity because they were cheap and convenient. But in time, highly successful marketing by food manufacturers and veterinary professionals who sell their products have led to the widespread belief that a commercial food is also the best way to provide a healthy diet. If you're like most caregivers, you probably feed, or have fed in the past, a canned food or kibble because you believe in your heart it's the right thing to do for that furry friend you care so much about. Unfortunately for our canine and feline friends, those packaged foods are not as nutritious as you might expect.

It's true that there are reputable companies that strive to build good nutrition and quality into their products. In general, those are formulated to be "nutritionally complete" based on guidelines established by the Association of American Feed Control Officials (AAFCO), an organization that establishes nutritional and labeling guidelines for animal food manufacturers. Many of those food labels also state they've been formulated and approved by a veterinarian.

So if you've been feeding a commercial dog or cat food that's made by a company you trust, and it meets all AAFCO guidelines, what's the problem?

Actually, there are a few problems. In brief:

- The food is highly processed.
- It's not fresh.
- The quality of ingredients is questionable.
- It may be "nutritionally complete," but for whom?
- It lacks variety, which can lead to deficiencies, imbalances, food sensitivities, and allergies.

Let's take a closer look at each of those concerns.

It's Highly Processed

Commercial foods are designed for convenience and longevity—convenience for you, longevity for the product (so it can sit on your grocer's shelf until you bring it home and feed it). Whether you prefer to open a can or scoop out a serving of kibble, it takes a good deal of processing to create food that is consistent from one package to the next, and that remains edible for weeks or months or more. Canned foods are subjected to extreme heat, so they can remain on the shelf without spoiling. Most dry foods are manufactured using extrusion, which uses high heat as well as pressure to create the uniform bits of kibble you find in the bag.

At high temperatures, many of the nutrients in food break down. Vitamins, enzymes, phytonutrients such as antioxidants and anthocyanins, and even proteins are damaged, so that much of the nutritional value of the original food is lost. Have you ever wondered why most packaged food labels include a long list of added vitamins on the list of ingredients? Those are added to replace nutrients that are lost in the manufacturing process—otherwise the food would not meet AAFCO's nutritional standards. Wouldn't you rather have your dog or cat get her nutrition from real food, rather than a laundry list of supplements?

And besides, those supplements added to packaged foods represent only the nutrients listed on AAFCO's guidelines—just the vitamins and minerals we know for sure are necessary for good health, based on current science. They don't begin to replicate the thousands of micronutrients that are available in fresh, unprocessed foods.

But there's another reason to be skeptical. Nutritional science has come a long way in recent years, and new discoveries are being made all the time. At this point, though, we have barely scratched the surface when it comes to understanding the vast array of vitamins, antioxidants, enzymes, and other natural components present in fresh, whole foods. So far, we've identified about 10,000 of these phytonutrients—those are the chemicals that plants create naturally to protect themselves from disease and other threats, and that also help us stay healthy when we eat them—and there are thousands more that are unknown. Most break down when exposed to high temperatures. You can see why it's impossible for any manufacturer to replicate the array of valuable nutrients that are lost when foods are processed into kibble or canned food, no matter how many supplements it adds. That means

why micronutrients matter

Most of us are aware of the importance of balancing "macronutrients" like protein, carbohydrates, and fats when we create a healthy diet. We're also familiar with "micronutrients," such as vitamins C and E and minerals like calcium, that are so essential for the body to function normally. But there are literally tens of thousands of micronutrients, including the valuable phytonutrients that come from plants, many of which are known to play important roles in keeping us—cats, dogs, and humans—healthy due to their anti-inflammatory, antiviral, and antioxidant effects, among others. There's still a great deal we don't know about these naturally occurring chemicals. But a growing body of research demonstrates that they protect us from many of the conditions that lead to early death or interfere with quality of life, including cancer, heart disease, stroke, diabetes, degenerative neurological diseases, obesity, and even premature aging.

your sweet friend loses the opportunity to enjoy the health benefits of those nutrients if his diet is based on commercial food rather than fresh, whole, home-prepared ingredients. (For more on this, see "What Would You Rather Eat?" on page 31 in Chapter 5.)

It's Not Fresh

The nutrients in any food degrade over time. We've been hearing a lot recently about the value of eating "farm to table"—that is, consuming our food as soon as possible after it leaves the farm. It's a great idea, because that's when food is at its best—it's most flavorful then, but also most nutritious. The healthy vitamins, antioxidants, and enzymes in any food are most abundant when that food is fresh off the vine, as they say.

The packaged food you buy today for your dog or cat is anything but fresh. It may have been made months ago, or longer, and there are few controls regarding how the food is handled between the time it leaves the factory and when it arrives in the store. Many are not even marked with a "Best by" date, so you have no way of knowing how old it is. So not only has the food lost nutrients due to processing, it loses even more nutritional value because it's…well, it's just old. Even if you choose a food that appears to contain pieces of vegetables or chunks of meat, it's inevitable that whatever nutrition was in the package when that label was applied has deteriorated by the time you feed it. You may not be able to grow ingredients for your pup or kitty's meals in your backyard, but if you buy the freshest foods you can find at your local grocer or farmstand, you'll increase the chances he's getting the best of what those fresh ingredients have to offer.

Food allergies, gastrointestinal troubles, and thyroid disease appear to be increasing in both cats and dogs, and some feel that repeated exposure to the wide variety of chemicals present in many commercial foods may be a contributing factor. Daily bombardment of your companion's system may damage cells, perhaps even creating a greater risk of cancer.

The Quality of Ingredients Is Questionable

Sometimes it feels like you need a degree in organic chemistry to understand the label on your dog or cat's food. Is that name you can't pronounce a vitamin or a preservative? What's the difference between chicken meal and chicken by-product meal? (Hint: "By-products" are parts of the chicken you and I would be unlikely to eat.) Does an ingredient called "meat" come from a cow…or some other animal you don't want to feed to your friend?

what's in a name?

The companies that sell packaged foods are always looking for new ways to market their products, and staying on top of current trends is an important part of that effort. As caregivers have become more concerned about the quality of ingredients, some manufacturers choose to change the way they label questionable ingredients rather than replace them with better-quality, more costly ones. For example, you might be reluctant to buy a food that contains "by-products." But instead of eliminating those and replacing them with human-grade foods, manufacturers have started calling them "upcycled" ingredients. Sounds better, doesn't it? Unfortunately, it doesn't mean they're any more desirable for you or for the family member who might have to eat them.

If the packaged food you buy does in fact meet AAFCO guidelines, it means the manufacturer claims to provide minimal levels of certain nutrients. But there's no guarantee where those nutrients come from. It helps to read labels, to be sure. But information about quality isn't on the label, and few manufacturers are willing to share much detail with you. Besides, wording can be tricky, and regulatory guidelines aren't as stringent as they are for human food labeling. Also, keep in mind that much of what appears on the label was put there by the company's marketing team. As you can imagine, marketing is one thing—performance is another.

Sadly, many of the ingredients that go into the food most caregivers rely on to keep their beloved dogs and cats healthy are things no one would consider part of a high-quality meal. The food may have the recommended level of protein, but the protein may be from a "dead, down, or diseased" animal deemed unfit for human consumption. It might even come from rendered animals—including those who have been euthanized.

Equally troubling are the artificial chemicals that are often added to packaged foods. Artificial flavors are added to replace the flavor that's lost in processing, so your friend will be willing to eat what's left. Artificial colors are there to make the food look appetizing to you, so you can feel good about feeding something that looks like real food. Preservatives reduce spoilage, and manufacturers still use chemicals for this purpose, including BHA, BHT, ethoxyquin, nitrates or nitrites, sodium hexametaphosphate, and others. Many of these substances are known carcinogens, or can lead to liver or kidney failure or other serious health problems.

what you see on the label may not be what you get

In January 2023, the American Chemical Society published a study conducted at the University of New Mexico that analyzed the DNA in six brands of commercial dog food. The study found that four of the six foods did not contain key ingredients—salmon, sweet potatoes, and beets—that were listed on the label. Perhaps more troubling is that each of the six brands contained DNA from at least twelve and as many as seventeen species that were not listed on the label—including dogs and horses.

It May Be "Nutritionally Complete," but for Whom?

Finding a way to feed balanced, nutritionally complete meals is perhaps the greatest challenge you face in your effort to provide good, healthy food for your beloved cat or dog. Even with all the drawbacks we've explored so far, a packaged food produced by a reputable company might appear to give you the best chance of providing optimal nutrition.

But the truth is, the best "nutritionally complete" food on the market is highly unlikely to be 100% nutritionally complete for *your* dog or for *your* cat.

How is that possible?

There are four key reasons why you should never count on a commercial food to meet your friend's nutritional needs as it claims to do.

> "The truth is, the best 'nutritionally complete' food on the market is highly unlikely to be 100% nutritionally complete for *your* dog or for *your* cat."

- AAFCO standards are based on a flawed system.

- Nutrition is an evolving science, and we don't know what we don't know.

- Every animal's nutritional needs are unique.

- Each animal's nutritional needs change over time.

Let's take a closer look.

AAFCO standards are based on a flawed system.

The American Association of Feed Control Officials, or AAFCO, sets standards for measuring the nutritional adequacy of animal foods, and evaluates how well commercial products measure up. There are three ways commercial manufacturers can substantiate the quality of their dog food relative to AAFCO standards. The first is to pass a feeding trial approved by the association. The trial is performed in a laboratory, and assesses how acceptable the food is to dogs and cats and whether it provides the proper level of nutrients to prevent deficiencies.

Sound good? Perhaps. But who runs the trial? Most often it's handled by either the dog food company or an outside contractor that reports to—and is paid by—the company. A conflict of interest could affect the data, especially since some of the criteria are very subjective when it comes to symptoms of deficiencies. Another flaw is the length of the trials. Certain deficiencies, vitamin A for instance, may not show up for months, well after the trial is over. And what may be fine for one dog or cat, day after day, year after year, could lead to serious deficiencies in an animal with a different metabolism or genetic make-up. There have been tragic cases of heart problems as a result of some cats consuming the same brand of food for a number of years. Even though the product passed the criteria for "complete and balanced," these animals suffered, and some died as a result.

"AAFCO standards are minimal at best. If you intend to feed a diet that supports optimal health and longevity, you'll want to look beyond minimum standards for nutritional adequacy."

Another way to receive AAFCO's approval is to formulate a diet that meets their minimum and maximum nutrient levels on paper. These standards offer a lot of leeway to the manufacturer, and are designed to be adequate for the "average" animal, but they may not be optimal for your companion. In addition, there may be bioavailability issues, which means you can't be positive that the nutrients in the bag are actually getting into your friend's system in adequate amounts.

Some companies meet AAFCO's requirements through a sort of back-door policy. If they have one diet that has been approved through feeding trials, they can formulate a new diet that on paper is similar to their other product, and get the green light that way. The bioavailabilty of the nutrients could be all over the map, but the stamp of approval still applies.

The label on every bag or can of food you buy should contain a statement of nutritional adequacy, but beware of wording that can be downright misleading. For instance, most veterinarians think labels bearing the words "animal feeding tests" are still the best choice, but be aware that the fine print may indicate the food is only *comparable* to a diet that has been through feeding trials. If the label says "intended for intermittent or supplemental feeding only," it means there is no data to show that this food is balanced to meet your dog's needs—and it probably isn't.

Most important, keep in mind that AAFCO standards are minimal at best. If you intend to feed a diet that supports optimal health and longevity, you'll want to look beyond minimum standards for nutritional adequacy.

Nutrition is an evolving science, and we don't know what we don't know.

Every week, it seems, a new study emerges revealing new information about how diet affects good health. How much protein is enough—and how much is too much? Are high-carbohydrate foods bad for dogs and cats—or are they an important source of valuable nutrients? Which micronutrients can their bodies manufacture, and which ones must they get from food? What is the role of intestinal bacteria in immune response, cancer prevention, and the aging process? What phytonutrients should we be feeding to help them live healthier, happier, longer lives?

Expert opinions vary on all these questions and many others. What we thought we knew a few years ago now looks less certain, and in some cases has been proven flat-out incorrect. And yet, AAFCO guidelines, which have become the gold standard for commercial foods, are based on this uncertain and ever-changing knowledge base.

It makes sense, of course, to do our best to create a healthy diet based on the information we have available today. But it also makes sense to find ways to reach beyond the current information—and its limitations—to create a feeding strategy that protects against those gaps in our knowledge. That's exactly what the Fresh & Flexible meal plan is designed to do for you and your companion.

Every animal's nutritional needs are unique.

If you've ever had multiple dogs or cats in your home at the same time, chances are you've noticed that they don't all need the same amount of food, even if they're the same size. Some even seem to do best on one brand of food while others do better on a different brand.

That's because no two animals have the same nutritional requirements, even among animals of the same breed of the same species. Differences in metabolism, in the way they process foods and utilize certain nutrients, and even genetic factors are among the many reasons the diet that's right for one may not work well for another.

How is it possible, then, that adhering to a single set of nutritional guidelines, like those set by AAFCO, could ensure that every animal will get all the nutrients she needs, in the amount she needs them?

It isn't. In fact, the likelihood that your dog or cat is getting the best possible nutrition—*for him or for her*—from that packaged food is very low. That's true of the macronutrients, like protein, carbohydrates, and fats; it's also true of the thousands of micronutrients, like vitamins, minerals, and other phytonutrients, many of which are yet to be well understood by even the best veterinary nutritionists.

> "No two animals have the same nutritional requirements, even among animals of the same breed of the same species."

It's troubling. And the problem is made worse by the fact that we've been told to find a high-quality food and feed that food every day, for weeks, months, and even years. Imagine the consequences if that food does not provide one or two or three or more key nutrients in the amount your friend needs, as is likely to be the case. It's easy to see how deficiencies can occur, some of which can lead to illness or premature aging. In any case, it's not a good strategy for optimizing the health and longevity of someone you love.

Each animal's nutritional needs change over time.

Have you ever noticed that your dog or cat's nutritional needs seem to change as she ages? Just like humans, many senior nonhuman animals need to eat less food to avoid gaining weight, due to changes in activity level and in the way their bodies process food. Often, older individuals' protein needs change. Some need more protein to stay healthy, while others may need to restrict protein levels to protect kidney function. Regardless of her age, your friend's nutritional needs change during times of stress; her body may require more calories than usual, and certain vitamins are more likely to become depleted.

The needs of any given animal change over time due to changes in health, environmental stress, activity level, and age. How, then, is it possible that a single packaged food can be "nutritionally complete" for every dog or cat, or even for most of them, for months and years on end?

To be sure, even with all their limitations, the AAFCO standards have their place. Choosing a food that's based on an established set of nutritional guidelines is a useful starting point, as it protects you from buying a food made from little more than fillers and artificial flavors. But it simply can't be seen as more than a baseline for quality, and you want much more than that for everyone in your family, including—especially?—your cat or dog. Don't allow that single parameter to give you a false sense of certainty that your friend is getting everything she needs. It's simply not a guarantee that that's the case.

It Lacks Variety

As worrisome as are all the issues we've discussed so far, the practice of feeding the same food every day makes them worse. If there are any shortcomings in the food you choose—and as we've seen, it's likely there are—those shortcomings will be amplified over time, and your companion's ability to thrive will become more and more diminished. They may even cause her to develop serious health problems. Even if you're meticulous about your research and find the best kibble or canned food on the market, if it contains more protein than she needs, or lacks a sufficient amount of a vitamin or mineral to meet her unique requirements, any problems will be amplified the longer she relies on it as her primary source of nutrition.

Eating a food that meets most but not all of her needs for a few days is unlikely to make her sick. But if she eats that same food for weeks and months, any deficiencies or imbalances will be compounded. That's when her quality of life may be seriously impacted.

And when your friend is exposed to the same food day after day over an extended period of time, it increases the likelihood she'll develop food sensitivities or allergies.

For all of these reasons, it's clear that for any diet to be truly healthy, it must include one essential ingredient: variety. That's the best way to avoid deficiencies and imbalances, food sensitivities, and allergies. Sadly, before the introduction of the Fresh & Flexible meal plan, variety was almost never included in dietary recommendations for our companion animals. Fortunately for those you feed, that's about to change.

We'll explore this in more detail in Chapter 4, "The Single Most Important Ingredient in a Healthy Diet." For now, keep this in mind: If you've been feeding the same packaged food for longer than a week, now is a good time to make some changes.

chapter 3

A Home-Cooked Recipe Doesn't Solve the Problem

Maybe you've already had concerns about packaged foods. Several have made headlines in recent years as the subject of recalls due to serious health problems some animals have suffered due to contamination or harmful additives. And with the growing awareness of the benefits humans experience when they eat fresh, whole foods, versus the harmful effects of highly processed foods, many caregivers have decided it makes sense to feed home-prepared meals to everyone in the family—including their cats and dogs.

Most often, though, that decision leads to uncertainty about what to feed, followed by a search for a tried-and-true formula: a recipe. A quick online search yields a long list of articles and books that offer tasty-sounding recipes; some have even been formulated by trained veterinary nutritionists. You choose one, or maybe two, add the ingredients to your grocery list, and set about cooking up a pot of homemade cat or dog food for your sweetie.

If that sounds familiar, you've done a great job of going the extra mile in your commitment to create a healthy diet. If the recipe you're feeding has been well-designed to meet known nutritional requirements, and you're using fresh, whole ingredients to prepare it, your friend is probably better off than if he were eating a packaged food. You've eliminated three of the five concerns we've raised about commercial foods:

- Your home-prepared food is not highly processed.

- The meals contain only fresh, whole foods.

- You know exactly what's in the bowl—no by-products, no artificial flavorings, colorings, or preservatives, and no contaminants.

Unfortunately, it still falls short. A home-prepared diet based on a well-designed recipe is good—and likely better than any packaged food you can buy—but it's unlikely to meet all your companion's unique nutritional needs. That because the best recipe out there doesn't address the other two concerns we discussed in Chapter 2:

- Even if the recipe you use is designed to meet AAFCO guidelines to the letter, those guidelines cannot possibly address the exact needs of *every* individual, or of *any* individual throughout the course of a week, a month, or a lifetime.

- It lacks variety, which can lead to deficiencies, imbalances, food sensitivities, and allergies.

Let's take a look at how those issues apply to a home-prepared recipe.

"Nutritionally Complete" Is a Moving Target

Nutritional science is constantly changing. What we thought we knew ten years ago about canine or feline nutritional requirements has changed, and is likely to continue to change in the coming years as new research corrects the misinformation we're relying on now. What's more, no two animals are the same, and one individual isn't the same for long. It's easy to see that the dietary needs of an active Border Collie are different from those of a couch-potato Great Dane. But two cuddly tabby cats who look nearly identical are also unlikely to have exactly the same needs for every nutrient we know about, let alone those we've yet to assess. They may require different levels of micronutrients, or do best on different proportions of protein and carbohydrates.

And, as we've seen, when an animal eats the same food every day, all of these concerns are compounded. Any deficiency is amplified when there's no opportunity to erase it by eating something different tomorrow or the next day. A lack of variety

"A home-prepared diet based on a well-designed recipe is good—and likely better than any packaged food you can buy—but it's unlikely to meet all your companion's unique nutritional needs."

in the diet also means your friend is exposed to the same components day after day after day, which can increase the risk of developing food sensitivities or allergies.

There's no getting around it. Whether we're feeding commercial foods or a home-prepared meal, if we rely on standardized guidelines, formulas, or recipes designed to create a meal suitable for every animal, we'll miss the opportunity to provide optimum nutrition for each one.

There's another drawback to following a home-prepared recipe that's worth noting: It's probably the least convenient, most time-consuming way to feed your friend. You need to shop a whole separate grocery list just for your dog or cat, then cook extra meals on top of the meals you already cook for your human family members. How do you find time for that? And what happens if it's time to make dinner for your sweetie, but you discover you're out of a key ingredient—or two or three? Do you drop everything and run to the grocery store? I seriously believe your time and energy are too precious to spend so much of them shopping for and preparing a special recipe when that's entirely unnecessary—and doesn't even provide the best possible diet.

If the prospect of providing optimum nutrition has seemed daunting and exhausting up to now, take heart. It's far easier to do and less time consuming than you've been led to believe—we just need to approach feeding from a different perspective. The Fresh & Flexible meal plan does exactly that. And it offers you a way to provide home-prepared meals that's far easier than those recipes you've been following.

chapter 4

The Single Most Important Ingredient in a Healthy Diet

It's time to take a moment to discuss what I believe is the single most important ingredient in any diet. It's the easiest one to add to your feeding strategy, and it solves many of the problems we've explored in previous chapters regarding commercial foods and home-prepared recipes.

That ingredient is variety. Variety, variety, variety.

Why Variety Is So Important

When you or your dog or your cat eat the same foods every day, three things happen.

1. You may not get all the nutrients you need, because there is no combination of three or four or even ten foods that contains all the nutrients your bodies need, in exactly the right amounts.

2. You run the risk of developing food sensitivities or allergies, which may be triggered by exposure to the same proteins or other components day after day after day.

3. Your bodies are less able to adapt to changes in activity level or health status, stress, and age, because each of those changes leads to altered nutritional requirements. If there's no opportunity to derive different nutrients from a different set of food sources, it's more difficult for the body to adapt to its new circumstances.

Including variety as an essential component in your feeding plan solves all these problems.

It Offers the Best Opportunity to Meet All Nutritional Needs

Take a moment to think about the way you eat. It's my guess you're reasonably conscious about eating a healthy diet yourself. You aim to meet all your nutritional requirements, and probably succeed at that fairly well. You're probably familiar with the Recommended Daily Allowances (RDA) established by the U.S. Departments of Health and Human Services (HHS) and Agriculture (USDA), and might even use those to help inform your dietary choices. Does every one of your meals meet those RDA recommendations? Do you meet them all in any single day? Is there a recipe you rely on that's been designed to provide all the nutritional requirements identified by the RDA? If you knew of such a recipe, would you eat that every single day, for weeks or months or longer? Assuming you don't, do you ever worry that you couldn't possibly be eating a healthy diet without following such narrow guidelines?

> She may not get every nutrient in the perfect amount every day—in fact, she probably won't—but it doesn't matter, because tomorrow or the next day there will be something different in her bowl, so she'll be able to draw different nutrients from different ingredients.

Probably not.

Instead, I'm betting that your strategy for eating a healthy diet is based on eating fresh, whole foods, including lots of vegetables and fruits, with lots of variety. You don't worry about getting every nutrient in precisely the recommended amount each day, let alone at every meal, because you're confident you can get everything you need by eating good, wholesome food, something different every day. I'll go out on a limb here, and guess that you may not even know what the RDA is for most nutrients, let alone all of them. But that's okay, because you trust the ability of a varied diet of good quality ingredients to get the job done.

And you'd be right. In fact, you're doing a much better job of getting everything you need that way than if you followed a single recipe based on the RDA, and ate that every single day.

Here's the thing. Your dog or cat can do just as well eating the same way. That's what the Fresh & Flexible meal plan is all about. When you feed a varied diet based on excellent ingredients, your canine or feline friend will thrive just as you do. A feeding strategy based on that principle will meet his needs better than any single kibble or canned-food formula or home-prepared recipe.

Why does it work so well?

As we've seen, there is no single formula that is correct for every dog or cat, because each individual's needs are different. When you feed a single packaged food or recipe every day, there's a chance that some nutrient is missing, or it's not available in the ideal amount. But when you feed a varied diet, your friend has the opportunity to draw whatever nutrients she needs, in whatever amount she needs them, from the wide array of ingredients she finds in her bowl over the course of a few days or weeks. She may not get every nutrient in the perfect amount every day—in fact, she probably won't—but it doesn't matter, because tomorrow or the next day there will be something different in her bowl, so she'll be able to draw different nutrients from different ingredients. With a variety of foods to draw from, it all balances out over a short period of time. She'll get everything she needs by eating the same way you do:

- A varied diet,
- based on fresh, whole foods,
- something different every day or every few days.

It Reduces the Risk of Food Sensitivities

Even a high-quality ingredient can trigger a food sensitivity or intolerance if the body is exposed to it every day for an extended period of time. Feeding different foods every day or every few days decreases the chances your companion will become reactive to any single ingredient.

A Varied Diet Makes It Easy to Address Changing Needs

When you become accustomed to feeding something different every day, it will soon be second nature to modify what goes into the bowl based on your friend's changing needs. If your dog joins you on an extra long hike on an early spring day, you might increase the amount of protein in his dinner to help him recover. If a visit from your neighbor's dog makes for a stressful day for your cat, you might include kale or blueberries to help lower stress hormones and reduce anxiety. If your companion puts on a few too many pounds or faces a health problem, and as she ages, you can easily adjust the meals you feed to help her adapt. (For more details, see "Find the Right Balance" starting on page 63 in Chapter 8.)

Diarrhea? Gas? A Varied Diet Is Not the Problem

But wait—doesn't changing a dog's or cat's diet cause digestive upsets? Won't she get diarrhea? I know, that's a reason we've been told it's best to feed that same packaged food forever, and never ever to feed "table scraps." There's some merit to that note of caution, but only if you're determined to feed the same food and only that food forever—and we've already seen the problems with that strategy. Here's why those warnings have some basis in truth, why you can safely let them go, and why your companion will be healthier if you do

Our bodies are amazingly adaptive. They perform countless complex functions every minute, all finely attuned to their internal and external environment. For example, when your dog or cat eats a meal, her body responds by providing enzymes to break down the nutrients in that food into substances her body can use. Those enzymes are tailored to the ingredients in her food—some help digest proteins, others break down starches, and still others work on fats, sugars, and more. The friendly bacteria in our digestive tracts also adapt to the foods that pass through. That's because those bacteria also play an important role in digestion, so they, too, must be tailored to suit the foods we eat. Put simply, certain ingredients cause certain strains of bacteria to flourish, because they eat those ingredients and thrive.

When your friend consumes the same foods, and only those foods, over an extended period of time, her body makes the enzymes needed to digest the ingredients in it, and the strains of bacteria that feed on those ingredients become more abundant. At the same time, the body stops making enzymes that would digest food it never sees. And as you might guess, bacteria that require certain food to thrive will die out if those ingredients never pass through the intestines.

> "When you feed a variety of foods on an ongoing basis, your friend's body will have an array of enzymes and beneficial bacteria at the ready to digest whatever comes her way. She'll have the flexibility to process new and different ingredients easily and without digestive upset."

If you've been feeding the same food over an extended period of time, whether it's a packaged food or a recipe you prepare at home, it's true that your pup or kitty may experience some digestive upset, flatulence, or even diarrhea when you make an abrupt change. That's because the enzymes and intestinal bacteria needed to digest the new food are not present. In time, though, her body will adapt, and provide everything she needs to handle the new ingredients in her diet.

Here's the good news. When you feed a variety of foods on an ongoing basis, your friend's body will have an array of enzymes and beneficial bacteria at the ready to digest whatever comes her way. She'll have the flexibility to process new and different ingredients easily and without digestive upset.

Even better, she'll reap the benefits of being able to draw whatever nutrients she needs from a broad range of food sources to meet her unique and changing requirements.

chapter 5

A Better Idea

The Fresh & Flexible meal plan solves all the problems we've seen in the ways we've been taught to feed our dogs and cats. Our beloved friends are developing chronic illnesses at a younger age, and all indications are that diet is a factor. As we've seen, commercial foods and recipes for home-cooked meals are based on guidelines that can't possibly address the unique needs of the companion you care so much about, and they lack the quality or range of ingredients, or both, necessary for him or her to thrive.

The Fresh & Flexible approach is a common-sense way to apply basic principles of good nutrition to provide the best possible diet, based on the good, healthy food you eat yourself. It works because you know what good food is. After all, if a varied diet of fresh, whole, minimally processed foods is good for you, why would it not also be good for your nonhuman friend?

The truth is, the same principles you use to design a healthy diet for yourself also provide the basis of a healthy diet for your dog or cat. It's that simple. And that's what the Fresh & Flexible meal plan is all about.

> "The same principles you use to design a healthy diet for yourself also provide the basis of a healthy diet for your dog or cat."

Sadly, we've been receiving a very different message for too long. Since the advent of commercial dog and cat foods, caregivers have been made to believe that the only way to feed a proper diet is to let someone else make it. But if you eat a reasonably healthy diet yourself, you can easily learn to feed your companion a healthy diet. If you've been relying on processed foods yourself, the principles behind the Fresh & Flexible meal plan will allow everyone to begin the journey to better health together.

Choosing good, healthy food for your companion really is very simple.

- Good food is fresh food, so you'll feed the same fresh ingredients you eat yourself. That way you'll know exactly what's going into the bowl.

- Good foods are whole foods, so you'll select minimally processed ingredients, organic if possible.

- For each meal you'll include an ingredient that's a good source of protein, a complex carbohydrate, and add a fresh vegetable or fruit (or maybe both).

- You'll add a healthy oil and a nutrition booster to make sure you've covered all your friend's needs. You might also choose to add a supplement or two.

- For the next meal you'll do the same—but with different ingredients in each category. Leftovers are great, so if you made a big pot of beans or rice, it's fine to feed it for two or three days, then freeze the rest for a quick and easy meal in a couple of weeks.

- Most important, you'll incorporate lots of variety into your friend's meals, drawing from a broad range of healthy ingredients to feed something different every day or every few days.

That's about it, a very simple strategy for eating well and feeding well.

As you might expect, there are lots of ways to fine-tune your strategy, to make sure you're delivering the foods that make it easy for your friend to get the nutrition she needs. We'll cover all the details in Part II of this book, starting on page 37. Before you know it, you'll have the confidence you need to feed fresh, healthy food, with lots of variety, so your dog or cat eats just as well as you do.

what would you rather eat?

When I was growing up, my mother often fed my sister and me a popular flaked breakfast cereal called Total, because it was fortified to provide 100% of every nutrient recommended by the RDA. I've come to believe that feeding a high-quality commercial dog or cat food, one that meets AAFCO guidelines, is a lot like feeding Total. Both are highly processed foods, but they come with claims that all nutritional needs will be taken care of if you eat it—or feed it—every day.

Think, for a moment, about what it would be like to eat Total cereal for breakfast every day, day after day...and again for dinner each and every day. For months. Or maybe for years. I don't know about you, but after three or four days I'd be craving a piece of spinach or a piece of fruit. And I'd wish for something hot and fresh and delicious from my kitchen.

And yet, we've come to expect our animal friends to be satisfied with just that sort of diet. We even expect them to thrive on it—a highly processed food that claims to meet the minimal known nutritional needs of some generic, hypothetical animal, but only because a virtual laundry list of supplements has been added.

From that perspective, it's easy to see why switching to a diet based on a wide variety of fresh vegetables, fruits, and other whole foods is likely to lead to dramatic improvements in health, vitality, and longevity.

It will also lead to a cat or dog who is very happy when mealtime comes around.

What Can You Expect after You Make the Switch?

The first thing you'll notice is that your companion is very, very happy that mealtime has changed. If you've been feeding packaged food, he'll be thrilled to finally be able to enjoy the yummy foods that generate those wonderful smells coming out of your kitchen. If you were already cooking a home-prepared recipe, he'll love having new and different flavors and textures in his bowl each day. If you choose to share your meals (yes, you can do that—see "Share Your Meals" on pages 72-73), you'll make him happiest of all. After all, we all know there's no food as delicious as whatever is on *your* dinner plate!

the sweet smell of good health

Savannah was a sick and broken-hearted, 6-year-old Great Dane when I adopted her from our county's shelter. Her teeth and gums were in terrible shape, and her breath smelled like she had a dead, decomposing animal in her mouth. Within a week after coming home and starting on the Fresh & Flexible meal plan, that dead-animal smell was gone, and her breath smelled clean and healthy. Within a couple of weeks her gums had begun to heal, and after a few months most of the plaque on her teeth had receded.

More recently, I unexpectedly took in a lovely and much-loved Border Collie on a short-term, emergency basis while her humans were traveling. She had been eating a relatively good-quality kibble and a very high-end (that is, expensive), fresh-frozen commercial food designed to replicate "fresh food"; her sitter sent along a supply of both. She seemed generally healthy, but had what I would call "dog breath," and her coat had the distinctive "doggie

Expect Improvements in Your Friend's Health

Best of all, chances are you'll soon begin to see signs that your companion is getting healthier right in front of your eyes. It's very common to see improved vitality and well-being in just a few days. Within weeks, real health benefits emerge, with results that can last a lifetime. Here are a few of the changes reported by caregivers who have made the switch:

- Energy levels are more balanced—vitality improves in many animals, and some become less hyperactive.

- Mobility improves, including a reduction in age-related joint pain and stiffness.

odor" common to many canines. She had been through a stressful time, and her appetite was off; she wasn't interested in eating any of those commercial foods she was used to, so of course I began offering her Fresh & Flexible meals. It was easy enough to do—no special shopping required, I just shared with her the fresh, wholesome ingredients already in my refrigerator. She was only with me for five days, but by the time she went home her breath was sweet and fresh and that doggie odor was gone from her coat.

The way a dog or cat smells is an indication of how healthy she is—or is not. There's a common misperception that animals just smell bad, and that there's nothing to be done but try to wash it away. But an unpleasant odor is not normal. If your dog or cat has bad breath, or if you feel you need to bathe her because of the way she smells, you may see a big difference after a switch to the Fresh & Flexible meal plan. Soon you'll be able to rub noses with her without recoiling, and relish burying your face in her lustrous, sweet-smelling fur.

- The coat becomes softer, shinier.

- Skin problems are reduced or disappear.

- Breath smells fresher, and the condition of teeth and gums improves.

- Digestion improves—there's less flatulence, and the odor of stools is less offensive.

- Some behavioral issues improve.

- Anxiety and stress levels may be reduced.

- Overweight animals are able to lose pounds while still enjoying ample, satisfying meals.

We don't yet have studies to demonstrate long-term outcomes for animals eating the Fresh & Flexible way. But we do know quite a lot about what happens when humans eat a varied diet of fresh, whole foods, including plenty of fresh vegetables and fruits: In simple terms, the risk of many chronic illnesses is reduced, and longevity increases. There's no reason to expect a different result in our dogs and cats. And given what we know about the effects of certain phytonutrients and antioxidants on certain common canine and feline health issues, it's reasonable to expect a reduced risk of chronic problems such as diabetes, cancer, degenerative joint disease, kidney disease, Cushing's disease, and more. I've seen outcomes like these in my clients, and veterinarians who now recommend the Fresh & Flexible meal plan for their patients also report excellent results.

You'll Reap Benefits as Well

I'm happy to report that there are many rewards in store for you, as well, when you switch to the Fresh & Flexible meal plan. First, it's easier. Okay, nothing is easier than opening a can or scooping a serving of kibble out of a bag. But if you want your companion to enjoy the health and vitality that comes from a truly healthy diet, there's no easier way to achieve that than by feeding Fresh & Flexible.

- There's no recipe to follow. That means there's no worry about running out of the "right" ingredients to make your pup or kitty's meals. Just use the good, wholesome food you already have in your refrigerator and pantry.

- You don't need a separate shopping list for your dog or cat. You'll buy the same healthy foods for her that you eat yourself.

- It's not necessary to prepare separate meals for human and nonhuman family members. You can if you choose, but since you're all eating fresh, whole foods, why not let everyone eat from the same pot?

- Many caregivers—myself included—report that they eat healthier when they're feeding Fresh & Flexible to their dogs and cats. Sometimes we're more diligent about making sure our animal friends have the best ingredients on hand for dinner than we are for ourselves. But I bet you'll find that when there's something delicious and nutritious on the menu for your sweetheart, it's easy to let that be what's on the menu for you as well.

Perhaps the most valuable benefit is one that no one expects. Feeding this way deepens your relationship with your companion. As you plan and prepare his meals every day, you become attuned to his needs and his happiness in a different way. Your rhythms become more aligned. We'll take a closer look at this in the Epilog, "An Unexpected Benefit," starting on page 99. For now, just know that feeding the Fresh & Flexible meal plan will take you further down the road to health, happiness, and a meaningful connection between you and your furry best friend than you imagine it could. Just give it a try, and you'll see.

part two
Fresh, Whole Foods, Something Different Every Day

part two

chapter 6

A New Way to Think about Feeding

As we've seen, the Fresh & Flexible meal plan is the best way to provide your dog or cat with everything she needs to meet her unique nutritional requirements. It also happens to be the easiest. Never again will you have to scrutinize a long list of ingredients on a can or package of food. No more wondering or worrying about the quality of ingredients in your friend's food, because you selected them yourself, fresh from your local grocery store. And when you prepare her meals in your own kitchen, there's no need to follow a recipe, and no worries about running out of any particular item called for in a recipe. You don't even need to buy special groceries. You prepare your companion's food the same way you prepare your own, using items you already have on hand in your refrigerator and pantry.

I understand, though, that if you're accustomed to trusting someone else to formulate meals for your companion, it

> "When you include variety as the most important ingredient in a healthy diet, he'll get all the nutrients he needs over the course of a few days or weeks, the same way you do."

can be daunting to have virtually unlimited options when dinner time rolls around. But remember, this approach is based on simple, sound principles of a healthy diet that you already use when you plan your own meals. It's simply a matter of applying those same principles, along with the guidelines you'll find in the coming chapters of this book, when you plan and prepare a meal for your dog or cat. If you've been relying more on boxed meals and takeout for your own dinners, the instructions in this book will be a great way for you to learn how to eat healthier yourself—especially with the added motivation of helping everyone in the family get started on the road to better health through good food. It's just a matter of changing the way you think about what it means to feed your dog or cat a healthy diet.

Here are a few tips to get you started.

Feed the Way You Eat

Don't worry about AAFCO guidelines, or about meeting your friend's exact nutritional needs in every meal or every day. You don't use the USDA guidelines for human health to plan every meal you prepare for yourself, and that's fine. You choose a selection of foods you know to be healthy—a good source of protein, some healthy carbs, and lots of fruits and vegetables—and eat a nice selection of different foods from one day to the next. Over the course of a week or two, you can feel confident you're getting all the nutrients you need from that fresh, wholesome food.

That's how the Fresh & Flexible meal plan works. You'll create your companion's meals the same way you create your own. Remember that when you include variety as the most important ingredient in a healthy diet, he'll get all the nutrients he needs over the course of a few days or weeks, the same way you do.

Still feeling a bit uncertain? Don't worry. In Chapter 7, "The Fresh & Flexible Meal Plan," starting on page 43, I'll help you get started with lots of ideas about the kinds of food to put in your friend's bowl, and guidelines to help you decide how much of each one. In later chapters I'll show you some easy ways to customize the plan for your unique and special friend, tips for preparing ingredients so they're easy to digest, and shortcuts that will make it all even easier for you. I'll even help you find alternatives for those days when there just isn't time to cook—for anyone.

Stick to the Basics

You'll find as much detailed instruction as you need in the coming chapters, but remember, it all comes down to three basic principles:

- Excellent ingredients, chosen thoughtfully and prepared with love and care, are the foundation of a healthy diet.

- Feed fresh, whole foods, something different every day or every few days.

- Protein, complex carbs, fruits and vegetables, and—you know what's coming—plenty of variety are the ingredients you'll start with. Add in some healthy oils, some nutrition boosters, and maybe a supplement here and there, and you're all set.

Trust Yourself

I know you want only the best for the dog or cat you love so much. You go to a great deal of effort and incur plenty of expense to provide for her in the very best way possible. You've always chosen the diet that you believed was best for her, based on what you'd been told by sources you trust.

But veterinary nutrition is an evolving science; research continues to reveal new information, and there's still a great deal we don't know. And don't forget, some of the most widely accepted advice emerged due to trends and events that are based less on sound nutrition than on convenience, capitalism, and good marketing campaigns.

It's time to return to the most tried-and-true principles you know you can rely on. For too long, caregivers have been told we don't know how to put good food into a dog or cat's bowl unless it was formulated by someone else. Most of us have become so convinced that we don't know what a healthy diet looks like that we've resorted to feeding highly processed meals with ingredients we can barely identify or might never consider eating ourselves. And because we've been taught to be afraid to think for ourselves when it comes to choosing healthy food for our animal friends, we've limited ourselves—and

"You know what good food is. You know how to feed yourself and your human family members. With the Fresh & Flexible meal plan, you can apply that same knowledge to feed the canine and feline members of your family."

them—to the monotony of a single packaged food or recipe, day after day, for weeks, months, or even years.

And we did it all because we believed it was best for them.

I'd like to help you reclaim your confidence. I'll say it again: You know what good food is. You know how to feed yourself and your human family members. With the Fresh & Flexible meal plan, you can apply that same knowledge to feed the canine and feline members of your family. And they—and you—will be healthier and happier as a result.

It's time to open a new chapter (literally and figuratively) on a new way to provide excellent nutrition for everyone in your family—the Fresh & Flexible way.

chapter 7

The Fresh & Flexible™ Meal Plan

The key to preparing fresh, nutritious meals from a variety of ingredients is to give yourself the flexibility to put different foods in your cat or dog's bowl every day, or every few days. There's no recipe to follow—you simply choose healthy, nutritious foods, much as you do when you plan your own meals. The Fresh & Flexible meal plan is an easy, convenient way for you to prepare wholesome, home-prepared meals for your friend, using the same healthy foods you eat yourself.

Most important, it's the best way to ensure that your friend receives all the nutrients he needs for a long, healthy, and happy life. Let's review a few of the reasons why that's true:

- Each individual has unique nutritional needs, so there is no single formula that's right for every dog or every cat.

- If you choose a recipe to follow, no matter how much care went into formulating that recipe, it's unlikely to include precisely the right balance of each and every nutrient *for your dog or for your cat.*

- Even if it were to include everything he needs today, what happens next week when your dog comes home happy but exhausted after an extra-long romp on the beach, or when your cat begins to show the first signs

> "There's no recipe to follow—you simply choose healthy, nutritious foods, much as you do when you plan your own meals."

she's entering her elder years? Nutritional needs change from day to day and week to week, but a recipe does not.

- Just as troubling, if you choose a great-looking recipe and feed it every day, in time your friend will be at risk of developing deficiencies of ingredients not present in adequate amounts—*for him*—or sensitivities to foods he sees day in and day out over a long period of time.

For so many reasons, it just makes sense to feed your companion the way you eat: Most of your meals probably include some protein, a carbohy-

good diet, good health

As a consultant in holistic health care for nonhuman animals, I've become absolutely convinced that, next to a safe and loving home, nutrition is the single most important factor in the health of our dogs and cats. Time and again, before a homeopathic or herbal protocol is even implemented, companions begin to get well just from a change in their diet. Whether they suffer from lameness, skin trouble, behavioral problems, or digestive ills, or any of a host of other difficulties, switching to a varied diet of fresh, whole foods almost invariably makes them better. I'll even go so far as to say that many difficulties are resolved just from cleaning up the diet, without ever going on to a remedy or other treatment. I've come to believe that the toxic substances in commercial foods—even in "premium" brands—are major contributors to health problems. Feeding fresh foods based on a single recipe can create health issues as well. When we choose instead to provide a varied diet of home-prepared ingredients, we make an investment that returns enormous dividends in saved vet bills and in years of vibrant good health for our beloved companions.

drate, and some vegetables or fruit, and you rarely eat the same thing more than a couple of days in a row. That's a great starting point for nonhuman family members, as well. From there, you'll choose proportions of protein, carbohydrates, vegetables, and fruits that makes sense for him, then finish the meal off with some healthy fat, a few nutrition boosters (more about those on pages 55-56), and perhaps a supplement or two. Soon you'll be on your way to using the Fresh & Flexible meal plan, a feeding strategy that allows your cat or dog's body to choose the nutrients he needs from a wide variety of food sources.

It's Easier than You Think

If you're accustomed to feeding kibble or canned food, switching to home-prepared meals can seem daunting. I understand…the prospect of having yet another meal to prepare every day may seem like a lot to take on. But it really doesn't have to be a burden. Meeting your dog or cat's needs can fit seamlessly into your existing lifestyle—including your current shopping, cooking, and eating habits. Cooking for your companion requires only a minimal adjustment to your daily routine.

- **Use the food you already cook for yourself to create a diet that meets her needs.** As long as you're already eating a reasonably healthy diet, simply modify the proportions and add a few supplements to create nutritious meals for your friend, right from your existing shopping list—even out of the same pot of food you're simmering for your own dinner. If your own diet is more quick 'n easy than fresh 'n wholesome, this is an excellent opportunity to let your best buddy inspire you to make changes that will benefit you both.

- **Cook in large batches.** Prepare one-pot meals, in batches large enough to last several days. It doesn't take long to toss some lentils or tofu, rice or potatoes, and a vegetable or two into a pot. In less than an hour you'll have a tasty meal for your cat or dog—and for you, too, if she's willing to share. Refrigerate or freeze leftovers in single-serving containers for subsequent meals that will be almost as easy to prepare as opening a can of "that other food."

- **In a pinch, whip up some "furry-friend fast food."** Develop a repertoire of super-quick meals for days when you're particularly short on time, from staples you always have on hand. While they may not meet all her dietary needs in one meal, the wholesome ingredients will keep her healthy, satisfied, and energized. In the context of a sound dietary program, she'll thrive by drawing nutrients from a variety of foods over the course of several days or weeks. (See "Fast Food for Your Furry Friend" on page 61 for suggestions.)

- **If you need to, use a high-quality prepackaged food as an occasional back-up.** You may find it helpful to have a kibble or canned food on hand to use now and then for convenience, or to supplement your homemade meals until you gain confidence. Be sure to choose a food that is labeled "all natural"—that is, made with no artificial additives—and made with human-grade ingredients. Just resist any temptation to rely on it more than you must.

How to Feed the Fresh & Flexible Way

The chart on pages 48-49 is a handy summary of what goes into your friend's bowl, with guidelines for how much of each ingredient to feed. Keep that handy as you prepare his meals the first few times. Soon you'll become confident that you have the good sense and judgment to create meals that satisfy his palate as well as his nutritional needs. Then watch how he responds, and adjust proportions and ingredients as appropriate for his body type, his metabolism, his unique nutritional requirements, and any changes in his health or activity level. Keep an eye on his weight, his coat, his energy level, his mood, and his general well-being. (See "Find the Right Balance" on pages 63-68.)

The following guidelines for each ingredient will help you get started, and also provide tips for making adjustments as needed.

PROTEIN: Most animals do well on about 30-60% higher-protein foods by volume. Here's how that translates to what's in the bowl: For every 1 cup of food, ⅓ to ⅔ of a cup will be a protein-rich food. Cats generally

protein from unexpected sources

High carbohydrate foods such as wheat, oats, barley, and potatoes, actually provide a significant amount of protein. Even greens like kale and vegetables like broccoli supply substantial amounts of amino acids, the building blocks of protein, to help meet your companion's protein requirements. While a diet of these foods alone would be unlikely to provide adequate protein to meet a cat's needs, or those of most dogs, they do make a notable contribution.

need a portion at the higher end of that range, while most dogs do well in the middle or lower end. For your cat, you might start at about 50% to 60% of the higher protein food, for your dog about 30% to 45%. If your friend seems less active than usual, isn't thriving, her coat is dull, or she's just a little picky with her food, you can easily increase the proportion of protein. If she can't seem to sit still, or has more energy than she can manage, decrease it. If you're feeding a diet based on raw meat and bones, protein levels will automatically be near the higher end of the range, or higher; consider increasing the amount of carbohydrates or vegetables. High quality protein sources include:

- **Beans and other legumes**—Lentils (brown and red), split peas, adzuki beans, mung beans, and other small beans do not require pre-soaking, cook quickly and break down well, and can usually be fed whole. Larger, firmer varieties, such as pinto, soy, red, and garbanzo beans, should be puréed in a food processor or mashed after cooking. Cook beans thoroughly, until very soft, for easier digestibility. (See "Dried beans and other legumes..." on page 60 for tips on cooking a delicious, digestible pot of beans.) Canned beans are a convenient option, but may require additional cooking to soften. Tofu and tempeh, made from soybeans, are highly nutritious and easy to digest. Peanut butter is an inexpensive and convenient choice; almond butter is also a nutritious option. How-

The Fresh & Flexible™ Meal Plan

What kind of food?	How much?	Which foods are they?
Protein	30% to 60% of the meal (Higher proportion for cats, middle to lower for most dogs)	Beans, lentils, split peas, tofu, tempeh, seitan, nut butter, eggs, meat, fish (Be mindful of the high fat content in nut butters.)
Carbohydrate	30% to 60% of the meal	Rice, quinoa, millet, polenta, rolled oats, barley, buckwheat, whole grain bread, whole grain pasta, potatoes, sweet potatoes, winter squash
Vegetables and fruits	10% to 30% of the meal	Leafy greens, broccoli, green beans, carrots, Brussels sprouts, cabbage, cauliflower, tomatoes, bok choy, beets Berries, apples, citrus, kiwi, peaches (pits removed), bananas, watermelon
Fats	1 teaspoon to 1 tablespoon per day	Flax, olive, borage, canola, hemp, coconut, fish; ground flaxseeds
Nutrition boosters	Amount varies depending on the booster. See pages 55-56 for guidelines.	Spirulina or blue-green algae, nutritional yeast, fermented foods, probiotics, mushrooms, wheat germ, garlic, alfalfa, lecithin

The Fresh & Flexible™ Meal Plan

What kind of food?	How much?	Which foods are they?
Vitamin-mineral supplement	For dogs over 20 lbs, 1 tablet per day; for dogs under 20 lbs and cats, ½ tablet per day. If supplement is made from whole foods, feed every other day.	Human grade multivitamin-mineral supplement that provides 200% or less of human RDA
Calcium supplement (essential for animals on a meat-based diet; not recommended for vegan dogs or cats)	For adult dogs, 500 to 600 mg (½ teaspoon powder) per 10 to 15 lbs body weight per day; double for nursing moms and puppies.	Calcium carbonate, dicalcium phosphate; eggshells
Amino acids (recommended for some vegan dogs; see pages 89-90 for guidelines)	Feed according to label instructions, adjusting the amount in proportion to your dog's weight.	Taurine
Vegecat/ Vegedog* (ESSENTIAL for vegan cats; optional for vegan dogs)	If used, feed in place of amino acids and vitamin-mineral supplement. Feed according to label instructions.	This is a supplement formulated specifically for vegan cats and dogs.

*Vegecat and Vegedog are available from Compassion Circle at CompassionCircle.com Please visit Chapter 11, "Can Dogs and Cats Go Vegan?" starting on page 97, for additional information about feeding a vegan diet.

ever, due to their high fat content, nut butters may be best saved for an occasional fast-food treat. Avoid brands that contain added sugar, salt, or preservatives; if possible grind them yourself in the bulk section of your grocery store.

NOTE: Macadamia nuts have been linked to vomiting, weakness, fever, and muscle tremors, and should be avoided.

- **Seitan**—This minimally processed food is popular in Asian cuisines and among vegetarians due to its versatile flavor, chewy texture (similar to meat), and exceptional protein content; ⅓ cup prepared seitan may contain more than 20 grams of protein. You can prepare it in your kitchen sink by simply rinsing the starch and fiber from a high-protein wheat flour or adding water to vital wheat gluten flour, then adding season-

soy and grains are good food

Soy and grains have gotten a bad rap in recent years, so much so that labeling a packaged food "soy free" and "grain free" has become a marketing tool. But are they really bad for your cat or dog?

Over many thousands of years of domestication, both dogs and cats have evolved to thrive on a diet similar to ours, including our grains and beans. It's true that some animals have developed allergies associated with those foods. But in most cases that's more a result of eating the same packaged food day after day for months or years at a time than it is an inevitable result of eating the grain or soybean itself. Most any food your companion—or you, for that matter—eats every single day for an extended period of time can trigger an allergy or sensitivity. In fact, meat and other foods derived from animals are far more likely to be a cause

ings. Packaged seitan is a convenient addition to meals, but some contain high levels of salt or other additives, so be sure to check the label.

- **Eggs**—Raw eggs offer more nutrition than cooked, but may pose a risk of salmonella or other bacteria that may be harmful, particularly if your friend is very young, old, or weak. If so, cook eggs thoroughly.

- **Fresh, lean meats**—Chicken, turkey, lamb, venison, pork, or beef. Meat should be cooked, or at least seared on the outside to destroy salmonella, E. coli, and other bacteria.

NOTE: Since meats are relatively high in phosphorus, when they are your primary source of protein it's especially important to add a calcium supplement to ensure the proper calcium-phosphorus balance.

than plant-based foods. Whatever the trigger, this is one of the big problems with relying on a single packaged food—the ingredients never change. Most animals do very well eating grains and soy products as part of a varied diet: rice and tofu today, polenta and black beans over the weekend, wheat and garbanzo beans on Tuesday, barley and lentils on Friday.

There's no reason, then, to avoid including grains and soy as part of your friend's healthy, varied, home-prepared diet. And yes, whole grains are superior to refined versions. Similarly, whole soy, such as tofu, tempeh, whole soybeans, and some soy milk, are better choices than the highly processed soy isoflavones or soy isolates found in some processed foods. This is one of many cases where the principles you apply to choose healthy foods for yourself and your human family work equally well when you choose healthy foods for your best friend.

CARBOHYDRATES: About 30% to 60% of your dog's diet will be made up of foods high in carbohydrates.

- **Grains**—Rice, millet, barley, oats, and quinoa (technically a seed) are just a few examples, but there are many others. Scan the shelves of your grocery store for different grains you can use to bring more variety to your friend's meals. As with beans, cook your companion's grains a little longer than you might cook your own, to enhance digestibility. Rolled oats can be fed raw or cooked.

- **Starchy vegetables**—Potatoes, sweet potatoes, and winter squash are options that most animals love. Whole, fresh corn should be puréed to make it more digestible, however cornmeal or polenta (technically a grain, because it's harvested when the kernels are mature and dry) is a tasty alternative that, when cooked thoroughly, is easily digested.

- **Whole-grain breads, pastas, and cereals**—Convenient and easy to digest, these are great options for a quick meal. Check ingredients and avoid added sugars or preservatives.

VEGETABLES: About 10% to 30% of your dog or cat's diet should consist of fresh vegetables. Serve raw or lightly steamed. Light cooking makes them easier to digest, but too much cooking destroys nutrients. Add the cooking water to your friend's meal for a little extra nutrition. Different colored vegetables contain different antioxidants and phytonutrients, so try to feed all the colors of the rainbow.

FOODS TO AVOID
Fried, processed, chemical-laden foods
Onions in any amount for cats, or in large amounts for dogs
Pork fat (bacon, fat from pork chops, ham)
Grapes and raisins (until further studies indicate they are safe)
Macadamia nuts
Chocolate

- **Green, leafy vegetables**—Spinach and leafy chard can be fed raw, finely chopped or puréed. Once chopped, raw greens tend to spoil quickly, so if you prepare a few days' meals ahead of time, add raw greens just before serving. Dense greens, such as kale and collards, should be lightly steamed. Any dark green, red, and purple vegetables will add an abundance of vitamins, antioxidants, and other phytonutrients.

- **Cruciferous vegetables**—Examples include broccoli, cabbage, Brussels sprouts, cauliflower, chard, kale, and bok choy. Most can be fed raw, if finely chopped, but some nutrients in broccoli and Brussels sprouts are more bioavailable if lightly steamed. Their antioxidant properties have been linked to a lower incidence of cancer in humans, however studies show that cooking reduces the cancer-fighting properties. Get the most from these vegetables by feeding them raw on some days, cooked on others.

- **Green beans**—Many animals consider these a favorite, tasty addition to their meals. They can be fed raw or cooked.

- **Tomatoes**—Cooked tomatoes and tomato sauce are especially high in cancer-fighting lycopene, an antioxidant with twice the power of beta-carotene.

- **Summer squashes**—Zucchini, crookneck, and starburst squashes. They should be lightly steamed or shredded to enhance digestibility.

- **Root vegetables**—White parsnips, purple turnips, red beets, and orange carrots are rich in antioxidants and other phytonutrients and provide plenty of fiber. Although best if lightly cooked, they can also be fed raw, but should be finely diced or shredded to enhance digestibility.

NOTE: Avoid feeding onions to cats, as onions have been linked to Heinz-body hemolytic anemia due to a compound in the onion that contains sulfur. Large dogs may be able to eat small amounts of onions from time to time, but caution should be used. Although they, too, are at risk of severe anemia, evidence suggests that a fairly large amount of onion must be consumed by a dog before any symptoms appear.

FRUITS: If your friend is unaccustomed to eating fresh fruit, she may be reluctant at first and need a little coaxing. It's well worth the effort, though, as she will benefit from the many vitamins and antioxidants in plump blueberries, a banana, or a fig, while crunchy apples and pears exercise and clean the teeth and gums. Fruits can be fed as a treat or added to a meal. Here are a few notes of caution:

- Reports from a national poison control center indicate that grapes and raisins have been associated with acute kidney failure in a number of dogs, and there are anecdotal reports of illness in cats. Until conclusive studies are done, it's best to avoid sharing these with your friend.

- Be sure to remove the pits from stone fruits, such as peaches, plums, or nectarines, as the jagged edges may be harmful to teeth and gums.

- If your companion is diabetic, the amount of fruit should be limited.

FATS: 1 teaspoon to 1 tablespoon of oil per day, depending on your friend's size and weight; use less if she is overweight, more if she has a health concern that would benefit from additional amounts. Meat-based diets usually contain adequate fat, but supplementing with plant-derived oils promotes optimal health. Choose flaxseed, canola, olive, borage, coconut, or hemp. Ground flax seeds are a fresh and healthful alternative.

NOTE: Use fish oils with caution due to the risk of toxicity in fish.

a note about organics

Even the freshest foods may contain residue of chemical pesticides, herbicides, and fertilizers, as well as hormones and antibiotics in the case of meat, that are used in the growing process. Many crops are grown from genetically modified organisms. Organic foods have been raised without these potentially harmful substances, and without genetic engineering. While the cost of organically grown ingredients is often higher than their commercially produced counterparts, their nutritional value is greater, and their purchase supports farming practices that are less damaging to the ecosystem. If you share your friend's organic meals, you'll probably find they taste better, too!

NUTRITION BOOSTERS: Augment your dog's diet with the vitamins, minerals, antioxidants, enzymes, and other nutrients provided by these high-powered whole foods. They contain an array of substances that work synergistically, so that nutrients are more easily assimilated into your dog's body. **Feed 1 or 2 nutrition boosters at a time, rotating through the list on a daily or weekly basis.** If your companion has a particular dietary need, you can provide at least a portion of his requirement by using one of these whole foods in addition to, for example, a supplement or vitamin tablet.

NOTE: Recommended amounts listed below may be fed "per meal."

- **Spirulina (blue-green algae)**—A true "super food," spirulina is an abundant source of minerals, including iron, as well as B-vitamins including B_{12}, chlorophyll, superoxide dismutase (SOD), and other antioxidants; also very high in protein, with 4 grams per tablespoon. Available in tablets or powdered form. **Feed about ¼ teaspoon per 30 pounds body weight.**

  NOTE: Some strains have been harvested from sources that are contaminated with heavy metals. Ask the manufacturer whether their source has been checked for contamination.

- **Nutritional yeast**—High in B-vitamins including B_{12}, as well as lysine and other essential amino acids, with 3 grams of protein in 2 teaspoons. It also aids in discouraging parasites. **Feed about 1 teaspoon per 30 pounds body weight.**

- **Probiotics**—Gut-friendly bacteria added to the diet help maintain and restore the intestinal flora, important for immune function and many aspects of good health; especially important for animals fighting an infection or those who have taken antibiotics. Fermented foods, such as sauerkraut or water kefir, are the best source, as they provide supportive nutrients and prebiotics along with many strains of friendly bacteria. **Add to meals in an amount appropriate for your friend's body weight.** Probiotic supplements provide specific bacteria strains, such as acidophilus, bifidus, and lactobacillus. **Follow feeding guidelines on the package, making proportional adjustments for your dog's body weight.**

- **Mushrooms**—There are many types of mushrooms that provide valuable immune support, and are an excellent source of important vitamins, minerals, fiber, and even protein. They also help maintain healthy intestinal flora. Shiitake, maitake, and lion's mane are delicious varieties that are well-known for their ability to protect against cancer. Cremini, portobello, chanterelle, oyster, and most other varieties are also excellent choices. Mushrooms must be cooked to be of nutritional benefit. They can be steamed, sauteed, or simmered in a pot of grains or beans **Feed about 1 to 2 teaspoons of cooked, chopped mushroom per 30 pounds body weight.**

- **Wheat germ**—High in vitamin E and many B vitamins; available raw or toasted. (Refrigerate, as it spoils easily.) **Feed about 1 teaspoon to 1 tablespoon per 30 pounds body weight.** Because it's high in fat, use with caution in overweight animals.

- **Garlic**—Stimulates the immune system and may help fight viral, bacterial, and fungal infections; has anti-inflammatory properties, and may help with joint pain. It also aids in discouraging parasites. **Feed about ¼ clove per 30 pounds body weight.**

- **Alfalfa**—High in minerals, particularly those that maintain the health of bones and joints; available in powdered form or as sprouts. **Feed about ⅛ teaspoon of powder per 30 pounds body weight. Add fresh sprouts to meals in an amount appropriate for your friend's body weight.**

- **Lecithin**—Aids in absorption of fat-soluble vitamins such as A, D, E, and K; supports mental alertness and helps correct some neurological problems. **Feed about ¼ teaspoon per 30 pounds body weight.**

VITAMIN-MINERAL SUPPLEMENT: Not required for animals eating a varied, whole-food diet made with organic ingredients, including nutrition boosters; recommended for all others, and for all seniors and those dealing with health issues. **For dogs over 20 pounds, feed 1 human multiple vitamin-mineral tablet (that doesn't exceed 200% of human needs) per day. For dogs under 20 pounds and cats, feed ½ tablet per day. If the supplement is made from whole foods, feed the above dose every other day.**

There are many vitamin supplements formulated just for dogs or cats, and even for animals at a particular stage of life. However, because of higher nutrient levels, a good multivitamin intended for human use is a better choice.

- As with any packaged food, read labels and avoid products that are made with artificial colorings, flavorings, or chemical stabilizers. **Avoid anything made with xylitol**, a common sweetener that is highly toxic to dogs and cats.

- Tablets made from concentrated whole foods are more likely to contain synergistically active ingredients, and are preferable to those that contain only isolated active ingredients.

CALCIUM: If meat is your main protein source, calcium is perhaps the single most important supplement for a successful meat-based, home-cooked diet. Even if you are feeding a variety of foods, in addition to meat, you'll need to provide an extra source of calcium to adequately meet your dog's nutritional needs.

- **Calcium carbonate** is routinely recommended by veterinary nutritionists, and it's readily available in most grocery stores and pharmacies. Feed a **600 mg calcium carbonate tablet (or ½ teaspoon of the powder form) for each 10 to 15 pounds of body weight daily for most adults, or 1 heaping teaspoon for each pound of meat; growing puppies and kittens need twice as much.**

- **Eggshells** are a form of calcium carbonate, and may be crushed and added to the meal as a convenient supplement. Cook the shells in a 350° oven for 10 minutes (or 1 to 2 minutes in a microwave) to kill salmonella and other bacteria; store in the refrigerator. One large, cooked eggshell provides roughly 2,000 mg calcium. **Feed ½ eggshell per 20 to 30 pounds body weight.**

- **Dicalcium phosphate** can be substituted in similar amounts, but should not be used if your dog or cat has kidney disease. The more bioavailable forms of **calcium marketed for human use** (gluconate, citrate, or coral calcium) should require lesser amounts to meet your dog's calcium needs.

If you're feeding a vegan diet that includes good amounts of leafy greens and vegetables, you do not need to add a calcium substitute. In fact, adding calcium alone could create an unhealthy imbalance in the calcium:phosphorus ratio. **Vegecat should be given to all vegan cats,** in place of a vitamin-mineral supplement, as it is created specifically to meet their needs, including their need for calcium, so no additional mineral supplementation is needed. If you feel you need to add minerals to your vegan dog's diet, use the Vegedog supplement, formulated for vegan dogs, in place of a vitamin-mineral supplement. Both Vegecat and Vegedog include phosphorus along with calcium to help keep ratios within the recommended range. Both can be purchased online from Compassion Circle at CompassionCircle.com.

NOTE: Commercial dog and cat foods contain adequate or even excessive amounts of calcium and phosphorus, so if you feed *some* prepackaged meals,

the most common mistake

Feeding home-prepared meals based on a variety of ingredients is a pretty straightforward strategy, and most caregivers are excited about giving it a try. But I've found there are different ways to interpret what "variety" really means. The most common mistake people make when they begin feeding the Fresh & Flexible way is to put a variety of foods into a pot...and then put the exact same variety of foods into the pot the next day and the next. For example, they may choose five or six different vegetables, add two or three grains and a couple of higher-protein ingredients. Then they repeat the process using the same ingredients—that is, the exact same combination of foods—each time they prepare a new batch of food.

It's true that there's a nice variety of foods in that pot. But if you prepare meals using the same ingredients day after day, week after week, you'll essentially be creating a recipe. As we've seen, feeding a single recipe for an extended period of time is unlikely

you don't need to supplement as heavily. Many holistic vets recommend 1 heaping teaspoon of calcium carbonate per each pound of meat you add to the diet.

Making the Switch to the Fresh & Flexible Meal Plan

I'm often struck by how easily most animals make the transition to the Fresh & Flexible meal plan. It's a testament to how well suited it is to supporting their well-being. Their bodies know what good food is, and most often they adjust quickly to their new and varied meals.

to provide your friend with all the nutrients he needs and in the correct amounts. If that "recipe" is not formulated according to known nutritional guidelines, the risk of deficiencies or imbalances is even greater. That means your companion's health may be damaged due to a deficiency or imbalance in a key nutrient. As with any repetitive diet, there's also a greater chance he'll develop a food sensitivity or allergy to an ingredient he sees every day. (See Chapter 4, "The Single Most Important Ingredient in a Healthy Diet" starting on page 23.)

Feeding a varied diet means putting something different in your dog or cat's bowl every day or every few days. You only need one protein-rich food, one carbohydrate, and one vegetable or fruit, along with one type of oil, one nutrition booster, and any supplements you choose. **Then choose a different food from each category for the next meal or the next day.** That way your friend will get all the benefits of a truly varied diet—just like you do when you plan meals for yourself.

The following tips will help you—and your friend—get started, then make adjustments to meet the unique needs of your much-loved friend.

Start small. Most animals do fine when making the switch, even when it's done with no phase-in period. But to make sure you're both comfortable, it makes sense to introduce the new diet gradually, especially if you've been feeding a single packaged food for several months or longer. Begin by replacing 25% of commercial food with fresh foods, and increase the percentage of fresh food every 3 to 4 days.

Adjust the portion size. Home-prepared food has a higher water content than dry commercial food, so if you've been feeding kibble, you'll need to put a larger volume of food in the bowl. For every cup of kibble you eliminate, replace it with about 1½ cups of fresh food, whether it's pancakes or scrambled eggs, a hummus sandwich or a pasta salad, a meat and potatoes dinner or Chinese stir fry.

Evaluate your friend's condition as you go along, and note any changes. Is she enjoying her new diet? What are her favorite foods? How are her weight, attitude, skin, and coat? Adjust amounts and proportions of protein, carbohydrates, and vegetables as needed. (See "Find the Right Balance" on pages 63-68 in Chapter 8.)

Remember to add a nutritional booster to each meal, and if your friend is aging or dealing with health issues feed a vitamin-mineral supplement every day or two. If you're feeding meat be sure to add calcium. If your cat is vegan, be sure to add Vegecat, available at CompassionCircle.com.

Dried beans and other legumes are cheap and nutritious sources of protein. Smaller beans like mung beans, red lentils, adzuki beans, and split peas do not require pre-soaking, and break down well as they cook so they're easy to digest. Soak larger beans in well-salted water for 8 hours or overnight, then drain and rinse thoroughly before cooking. Add a potato to the cooking water to help absorb indigestible sugars that can cause gassiness. (Discard the potato—DO NOT feed it.) A strip or two of kombu seaweed added to the cooking water will help break down indigestible sugars and enhance flavor.

Cook beans and grains longer than you might if you were cooking just for yourself, to help make them softer and easier to digest. If you're sharing your meals, you can always remove a portion for yourself and other human fam-

FAST FOOD FOR YOUR FURRY FRIEND

Too busy to cook? Worked late last night and didn't have time to shop? You thought you had one more single-serving of your pal's food in the freezer, but now it looks like Uncle Ron must have eaten it?

Your home-cooked meal routine has become second nature, but every now and then you need to whip up a quick meal from scratch in a flash. Here are a few ideas that will let you light up those big, hungry brown (or green) eyes, even if your cupboard is down to the bare basics.

(Please keep in mind that the recipes that follow are not nutritionally complete on their own, nor are they intended for use on a daily basis. They're offered here as occasional choices within the context of a well-balanced, varied nutritional plan. All recipes have been taste-tested and approved by our eager canine and feline food editors.)

California Cuisine
Your pal will be the coolest pup or kitty in the county. Toss tofu with rolled oats or barley. Add the juice from the tofu to moisten. Stir in some chopped spinach leaves or alfalfa sprouts, or a sprinkle of spirulina.

Lunchbox Peanut Butter Sandwich
This one is really simple. Layer slices of whole-grain bread with peanut butter. Break the sandwich up and toss with plain yogurt and some fresh, diced apple or blueberries. That's it. You're ready to go.

Burrito Bowl
Open a can of refried beans (not the spicy kind, just beans and maybe a little oil), stir together with leftover rice or other grain, and add diced tomato and avocado. Olé!

My Dish Is Your Dish
This one may be the easiest of all—in fact, it may already be your go-to Fresh & Flexible strategy—but it does assume a certain level of healthful dining on your part. Simply share whatever you're eating with your buddy. If you've been following the Fresh & Flexible guidelines so far, you can be sure that if it's good enough for him, it's good enough for you!

ily members while the beans or grains are still firm and chewy. Then leave the rest on the stove until the skins begin to break down and they're a nice soft consistency.

Mash or purée larger, firmer beans, like garbanzos, black beans, or kidney beans, to make them easier to digest.

A big pot of stew can provide hearty meals for a few days now, and for next week if you freeze some leftovers. Choose brown rice, quinoa, or other grain; add mung beans, adzuki beans, lentils, or other beans, or meat. Near the end of cooking time stir in vegetables and a little garlic and olive oil, then continue cooking just until the vegetables are tender. Stir in fresh parsley or turmeric at feeding time. Add calcium if your stew contains meat.

Carrots, apples, and broccoli stalks make tasty snacks, help exercise your friend's teeth and gums, and satisfy her desire to chew.

When you first switch to a fresh-food diet, you may see pieces of whole, undigested foods appear in her stool. After a few weeks, you should see less food passing through. If not, try cooking those items a little longer, or purée them in a food processor or blender. Add digestive enzymes and probiotics to aid digestion until your friend's system adjusts.

If your companion is a little fussy, try a tasty topping to spark her interest. Try tomato sauce, nutritional yeast, spirulina, vegetable or coconut oil, broth, soy or dairy milk, butter (vegan or dairy), a sprinkle of vegan or dairy parmesan or other hard cheese. (Find more tips in "If Your Friend Has Discriminating Tastes" on pages 68-70.)

chapter 8

Modify Meals to Meet Your Friend's Needs

One of the great benefits of the Fresh & Flexible meal plans is that it's designed to meet the unique nutritional requirements of every dog or cat. When you first introduce it to your friend, and as her needs change over time, you can easily modify the meals to address the needs of each member of your family.

Find the Right Balance

As you've seen, the plan offers guidelines for how much of each component of the meal should go into the bowl—but it does not specify exact amounts. That's because the correct balance of ingredients is different for every animal. How will you know what's right for your friend?

Begin by feeding proportions within the ranges suggested in the Fresh & Flexible chart on pages 48-49. Then observe how he responds. By watching for simple clues, you'll know if you need to make any adjustments. Here's what to look for.

Energy Level

Most animals on the Fresh & Flexible meal plan exhibit a healthy, vibrant, balanced energy level. In fact, it's become a hallmark of dogs and cats who eat this way.

But if your companion doesn't seem to have as much pep as usual, or seems a little dull, it might mean he needs a different balance of higher-protein and carbohydrate foods. In most cases, increasing the amount of protein will put a spring back in his step. But for some, more carbohydrates are the answer. Try adjusting the proportions in either direction to see what gets the best response.

It might come as a surprise to learn that many animals get too much protein. It seems to be more of an issue for dogs than for cats, perhaps because cats generally have higher protein requirements than dogs. But so many of our canine friends are considered "high-energy" dogs—and while that's true of some individuals, and particularly some breeds, others might more accurately be called hyperactive or hypersensitive. Whatever the label, a dog who has too much energy is not at peace, and not as happy as any of us—including him—would like him to be. Here are some clues to watch for:

- Your dog is restless at home even after a nice long walk. He paces, as though looking for something to do, and has a hard time settling down to relax.

- When he's off leash, he seems to run as though he *has to* run, as though he has more energy than he can handle—not simply for the joy of running free.

- He exhibits inappropriate behavior, such as aggression or bullying other dogs; chewing on inappropriate objects; or chewing or licking his feet, limbs, or other body parts.

- He has trouble focusing his attention. Even though he enjoys playing games or learning new skills, he's easily distracted, and seems to have a short attention span. When on a walk, he's unable to walk calmly by your side, even though he's been taught to do so, and pulls on the leash or lunges at people or other dogs.

- He's often anxious, even when there's not an obvious reason to be (such as a thunderstorm or a trip to the vet).

Keep in mind that there are a number of factors that can cause these behaviors, and some have nothing to do with diet. But it's worth considering whether reducing the amount of protein in your dog's diet might make life more peaceful for everyone.

Skin and Coat

One of the first changes most caregivers see after switching to the Fresh & Flexible plan is a softer, more lustrous coat.

However, if after a few weeks on her new diet your friend's coat seems dull, or her skin is dry or flakey, try increasing the amount of fat. You can safely double the amount of oil recommended in the Fresh & Flexible chart on pages 48-49. Make sure you're rotating through a variety of different oils to make sure she's getting all the various fatty acids and other micronutrients she needs.

For some animals a dull coat may indicate a need for more protein. Try increasing the proportion of higher-protein foods in the bowl. Be sure to rotate among a variety of different foods—something different every day or every few days. Check her stool to see if any pieces of food are passing through undigested. If so, cook those foods longer or purée them for greater digestibility.

Appetite

It's rare to see a dog or cat who doesn't love having different fresh, home-prepared foods in her bowl every day. We all know that look that says, "Can I have some more, please?" and Fresh & Flexible dogs are masters at it. Even notoriously fussy cats often become much more enthusiastic when the refrigerator door opens.

But there's a difference between enthusiasm and being inordinately hungry. If your friend is hanging out in the kitchen when its hours before mealtime, or forgets to be polite and let your finish your meal in peace, or goes to unusual lengths to find food ("She never raided the trash can until now!"), she might not be getting all the nutrition she needs. Here are some likely solutions:

- She may simply need more food in the bowl. Keep in mind that fresh food has a much higher water content than kibble (or even some canned foods), so you'll need to increase the volume of food in the bowl by at least 25% compared to the amount of kibble she was eating before. In any case, the simplest and best solution to hunger pangs is often more food, so try that first.

- Make sure you're feeding plenty of variety. That doesn't mean putting a large number of ingredients into her bowl all at once, then feeding the same combination of foods for weeks on end. Nor does it mean feeding a different vegetable every day, but relying on the same carb (such as rice) or protein (such as lentils) at every meal. The Fresh & Flexible plan means choosing one higher-protein food, one carbohydrate, one vegetable or fruit, a healthy oil, and a nutrition booster or two for each meal—*and then feeding a different food from each category* every day or every few days. If you're not including that level of variety in your friend's meals, she may be missing key nutrients. That alone will cause her to feel more hungry than she should.

- Try adjusting the proportion of protein and carbohydrates in the bowl. Some animals need more protein to feel satisfied, others need more carbs. See what works best for your friend.

- Vegetables and fruits are the nutritional powerhouses of any diet, and they supply many of the essential micronutrients that are difficult to find in other foods. Make sure your companion is getting plenty of both—with lots of variety, of course. Remember, too, that a carrot or an apple, or any number of fruits and vegetables, make tasty and healthy snacks. That's a fun way to add more of them to everyone's diet.

Weight

One of the great benefits of the Fresh & Flexible meal plan is that it makes maintaining a healthy weight almost effortless, because it's so easy to modify meals to meet your friend's needs.

For those who are carrying a few extra pounds, weight loss has never been easier—or more painless. Simply reduce the proportion of higher-calorie foods and fill the bowl with healthy, low-calorie foods like vegetables and fruits. Your buddy will never feel deprived when his meals are just as ample as ever. And he'll get all the health benefits and enjoyment of eating all those delicious, nutrient-dense foods. (Of course, you'll also want to be sure he's getting all the exercise he needs.)

For those who need to gain a few pounds,

- Increase the volume of food in his bowl.

- Feed more frequently. The same amount of food divided into more frequent but smaller meals eaten throughout the day may allow your friend to digest it more completely, resulting in better nutrition and weight gain.

- Increase the amount of fat—within reason. Healthy oils are an essential part of any healthy diet, but too much fat can cause problems even for those who need to gain weight. Start with the guidelines in the Fresh & Flexible chart on pages 48-49, then increase it by up to twice the amount indicated.

- Increase the volume of higher-calorie foods in the bowl. Don't skimp on healthy vegetables and fruits. But higher-protein foods and carbohydrates are generally more calorie dense, so adding more of those will support weight gain. Some animals do best with a higher proportion of protein, others add pounds with more carbs. Try adjusting meals in both directions to discover what works best for your best friend. Don't forget to include higher-calorie foods like peanut or almond butter—just be aware of the added fat content they bring to the meal.

> "For those who are carrying a few extra pounds, weight loss has never been easier— or more painless!"

Health Issues

If your friend is dealing with a particular medical condition that requires reducing or increasing the amount of a particular vitamin, mineral, or other micronutrient, the Fresh & Flexible meal plan makes it easy to select foods that meet those needs.

For example, if your cat or dog is dealing with chronic kidney disease, your veterinarian may recommend a diet that's relatively low in phosphorus. Or if she needs extra immune support, you'll want to be sure she's getting plenty of antioxidants. You can address those needs simply by choosing foods that meet the nutritional profile you're aiming for. There are a number of websites and apps that provide detailed nutrition data for many foods. An excellent one is My Food Data, at MyFoodData.com. It also has a tool that shows you which foods are highest and lowest in a key ingredient.

If Your Friend Has Discriminating Tastes (a.k.a. "The Fussy Eater")

Most dogs and cats love finding fresh food in their bowls, and welcome the variety of flavors they eat from one day to the next when you feed the Fresh & Flexible meal plan—even when ingredients are simple, unadulterated, and straight from the farm, no fancy preparation required. But we all have our own preferences and relationships to different foods and flavors, and our dogs and cats are no exception. It's rare, but some animals are reluctant to try foods that are unfamiliar. Occasionally, a dog or cat who has been eating kibble for years has trouble adjusting to the array of new aromas, flavors, and textures that suddenly appear in his bowl. And even the most enthusiastic eater might become fussier when he's not feeling his best or as he ages.

If your dog or cat has a particularly discerning palate, here are a few strategies to help you entice him to learn to love his delicious, nutritious meals.

Give her a choice. Try separating items in the bowl rather than mixing them all together. Some animals prefer to be able to work their way through the different flavors. It also allows you to identify which foods your friend enjoys and which ones she avoids—and those may be the reason she rejected the entire meal. You can then plan future meals more suited to her taste preferences.

Add flavor enhancers. Sprinkle them on top, mix them in lightly, or add them before or during cooking. Sometimes that's enough to get him started on a meal, then he'll realize how tasty those fresh ingredients are and keep eating. Here are some favorites you can try:

• Oils – Instead of mixing his flax seed, olive, coconut, or other oil into his food, drizzle it over the top so he gets the full impact of the aroma and flavor.

- Nutritional yeast – Sprinkle it on top or mix it lightly into the meal, or add it during cooking. Dust his tofu with it before sautéing, or toss it with his vegetables before steaming.

- Garlic – It's perfectly okay to feed garlic raw, but fussy eaters may enjoy the milder taste when it's powdered or lightly cooked. Sprinkle it over the meal or add it during cooking. Garlic and nutritional yeast together add loads of flavor that most animals love.

- Spirulina – This dark green superfood is so nutrient dense that there are many reasons for animals to be drawn to it. It has an almost fishy aroma that's also enticing.

- Powdered kelp or other seaweed – Again, the briny, fishy taste makes it a popular choice.

- Tomato sauce – Cooked tomatoes add a light umami flavor, which may be a reason so many dogs and cats enjoy it.

- Yogurt – Most dogs and cats enjoy yogurt, including nondairy varieties like soy, cashew, or coconut. Choose a variety that does not contain added sugar.

- Peanut (or walnut or almond) butter gravy – This may not be part of your culinary repertoire—yet—but your dog or cat will thank you if you add it. It only takes a small amount of nut butter stirred into hot water to make a delicious topping that even the most discriminating eater is likely to enjoy.

- Soy sauce – But use it sparingly due to the high sodium content.

- Broth – Homemade or store-bought will do, but choose a no- or low-salt variety.

- Yellow foods – For some reason many cats love yellow and orange fruits and vegetables, such as corn, melon, sweet potato, and cooked carrots. It's not clear why, but it may be due to the carotenoids in yellow foods.

Show her how delicious it is. Most animals are delighted to eat whatever their human is eating, so use that to your advantage. Put some of your friend's meal on your own plate, then eat it with gusto—and as much drama as you can muster. Smack your lips, ooh and ahh over it, roll your eyes at how delicious it is. You might even offer her a sniff as you bring the food to your mouth, all the while telling her how wonderful it tastes. When she starts to look envious, offer her a bite or two, then continue eating it yourself. Carry on until she's convinced, then let her eat her meal from your plate, because…it just tastes better that way.

chapter 9

It's Easy and Flexible Enough to Meet *Your* Needs

Life is busy and time is short. If you're like many of us, there just aren't enough hours in the day for you to prepare a whole new set of meals for your dog or cat, in addition to your already-demanding grocery shopping, cooking, and clean-up duties. While you'd love to see your friend reap the nutritional benefits of the Fresh & Flexible meal plan, you might be struggling with the idea of taking on a lot of extra work. And in all honesty, it's probably not fair to ask you to. For a diet to be successful for your companion, it has to be successful for you as well.

But truly, feeding the Fresh & Flexible way is not a lot of work—or at least it shouldn't be. Cooking for your dog or cat does not have to be complicated or difficult or excessively time consuming. The hardest part is letting go of the idea that "dog food" or "cat food" is different from "human food." With the Fresh & Flexible plan they're all the same, so cooking for your pal is no more difficult than cooking

> "Good food is good food, no matter who is eating it. "

for yourself. It all comes down to changing the way we think about feeding our dogs and cats. Good food is good food, no matter who is eating it. And since there are no recipes to follow, there's no separate grocery list and no extra meal to prepare. You just use what's in the pantry and refrigerator to make a nice meal for yourself…but make a little more, so there's enough for everyone. If you prefer to eat foods you'd rather not share, that's fine, too.

Fresh & Flexible is so…well, flexible, that you can still adapt it to your existing cooking routine to minimize the amount of extra work you'll have to do.

Here are a few of the strategies I use to feed my own best friend the best possible diet with the least amount of work for me.

Share Your Meals

If you eat a reasonably healthy diet yourself, it takes very little additional effort to prepare meals for a canine or feline family member. You probably already build most of your own meals around a higher-protein food, a carbohydrate, and vegetables or fruit. As we've seen in the Fresh & Flexible chart on pages 48-49, that's also the basis of your meals for your dog or cat. Add some healthy oil to his bowl, stir in a nutrition booster, and add any supplements he needs (be sure to add a calcium supplement if he's eating meat, or Vegecat if your cat is vegan). That's it.

There are a few modifications you may need to make—but just a few.

- Onions are one of the few "human foods" that most dogs and cats should avoid. A large dog is unlikely to have a problem if he eats a small amount now and then, but they can cause hemolytic anemia in small or medium-sized dogs, and are especially dangerous for cats. If you enjoy onions, prepare them separately and add them into your meal after you've separated your portion from your friend's. Raisins, grapes, macadamia nuts, and chocolate should also be kept out of your dog and cat's meals.

- Minimize the use of highly processed or very fatty or fried foods, or those with excessive salt or sugar, and avoid anything with artificial flavors, colors, or preservatives. An occasional indulgence—within reason—probably won't do any harm in the context of an otherwise healthy, whole-foods diet. Just get back on track with clean, minimally processed ingredients for the next meal.

- Herbs and spices are a wonderful addition to any meal, and your dog or cat will enjoy the added flavor and health benefits they bring, just as you do. But if you also enjoy very *hot* spicy food, it's best to add those chili peppers after you've separated out a portion of the meal for your friend. While some seem to enjoy a little heat in their food, too much can cause a digestive upset or discomfort as it passes out in the stool.

- It's often helpful to cook beans and grains longer for your dog or cat than you might normally cook them for yourself. If you see undigested foods passing through in her stool, cooking those items longer will make them softer and easier to digest. Just remove your portion from the pot when the food is cooked to your liking, then leave hers to simmer a few minutes more. Or try mashing or puréeing her portion before adding it to her bowl.

- Avoid falling into a rut. If your go-to meal is pasta four or five times a week, or you find yourself relying on rice and lentils more often than you'd like to admit, remember that variety is the single most important ingredient in everyone's diet. Use the principles of the Fresh & Flexible plan to inspire you to choose different foods every day or every few days, so you, your dog, and your cat can all draw exactly the nutrients you need from a broad range of healthful ingredients. You'll join the ranks of the many caregivers who find they eat a healthier diet themselves when they begin feeding Fresh & Flexible meals to their furry best friends.

Cook in Batches

You know by now that eating a variety of foods is essential to a healthy diet. But that doesn't mean you need to eat—or feed—entirely different ingredients every single day. As long as there's something different on your plate or in his bowl every few days, you're covered. So whether you share your meals or prefer to cook separate foods for your companion, you can save time and effort by falling in love with leftovers.

When you make a pot of beans or roast some winter squash, or simmer up lentils and potatoes for a hearty stew, make enough for two or three meals. You'll enjoy being able to pull a tasty meal out of the refrigerator at a moment's notice. Just steam some vegetables or chop some leafy greens, add them to the bowl—and to your plate—and dinner's ready. Remember, too, that most of those foods freeze well, and are especially handy if you package them up in meal-sized portions. That way, you can minimize your prep time for many meals to come.

Get Creative with Healthy "Fast Food"

Strategies for simplifying home-prepared meals for your friend are all well and good, but there are times when even that isn't practical—like those days when you're dashing out the door and barely have time to throw a sandwich together for yourself to eat on the run. Or when you get home late, the leftovers have all been eaten, and you're too tired to cook a proper meal. When you have only yourself to worry about, you cobble together something quick and easy and call it dinner.

With the Fresh & Flexible plan, that can work for your dog or cat, too. A smear of peanut butter on good whole-grain bread, with maybe some blueberries or chopped apples in the middle, just might make for a quick but satisfying meal for whoever happens to be hungry. You'll find more suggestions under "Fast Food for Your Furry Friend" on page 61.

Apply the Fresh & Flexible Principles—Even If Cooking Is Not an Option

Now and then I speak with a guardian who really wants to feed what's best for her friend, but simply can't find the time or energy to make home-prepared foods. Maybe she Simply. Does. Not. Cook, and dines out or gets takeout for the vast majority of her own meals. Or perhaps she leans heavily on frozen or boxed meals when she does cook for herself at home. She might travel a lot, and relies on sitters who can't be counted on to make the extra effort. I once spoke with a very loving, dedicated dog mom who lived on the road in a small travel trailer with only a small hot plate for cooking; healthy, home-prepared meals just weren't an option for herself or her dog.

If commercial foods are the only option, you'll never overcome the limitations of feeding highly processed foods. But you can vastly improve the quality of your friend's overall diet by adapting two core principles of the Fresh & Flexible meal plan:

- Choose products made with the best possible, whole-food ingredients.

- Remember that variety is *still* the single most important ingredient in any healthy diet.

How are either of those possible when feeding commercial food? Here are a few tips.

Scrutinize Ingredients Listed on the Label

While the commercial foods themselves are highly processed, you can look for products that are made from minimally processed ingredients, with no artificial flavors, colors, or preservatives. Look for whole, human-grade foods rather than those identified as "meal" or "by-product." Choose products made with organic ingredients if possible. Explore vegetarian and vegan options to avoid the hormones, antibiotics, and environmental toxins present in meats used in many commercial foods.

Finally, while an expensive price tag is no guarantee of quality, inexpensive foods usually cost less because they use cheaper—and often inferior—ingredients. This is one time when bargain hunting might end up costing you a lot more in terms of your friend's health.

While feeding kibble or canned food is hardly ideal, being highly selective about which food you choose will help you provide the best available quality within the scope of a commercial diet.

Draw from Different Brands that Use Different Ingredients

It is possible—to some degree—to incorporate variety into your friend's diet, even if you must rely on commercial foods. Simply choose four or five different brands of top-quality food, then rotate between those several brands every day or every few days. That way you'll increase the likelihood that, over time, your friend will be able to draw the nutrients she needs from a variety of different food sources, and reduce the chance of triggering a food sensitivity or intolerance.

Please note that I recommend choosing several different brands of food—not just different flavors within a particular brand. Many manufacturers offer several different flavors in their line of kibble or canned food, each with a different key ingredient such as turkey, beef, chicken, fish, or maybe duck. But you'll notice that, in most cases, the only thing that changes is the first one or two or three ingredients—everything else on the list of ingredients is the same. So if you choose several different flavors from a single brand, with the exception of those few ingredients your friend will be eating exactly the same thing, day after day after day. That's not a varied diet.

However, each manufacturer develops its own formula, so the entire list of ingredients is more likely to be unique. For that reason, if you select four or five different brands of food, you're more likely to be providing more variety among all the ingredients that go into each one. (Beware of different brands that are owned by one large corporation—they might all offer the same formula under a different label. Once again, scrutinizing the list of ingredients is key.)

So take heart. If a varied diet of home-prepared meals just isn't on the table (so to speak) for you or anyone else in the family, you can make the best of the second-best option. And of course, any time you happen to cross paths with a stalk of broccoli or a plump blueberry, be sure to share it with your furry friend.

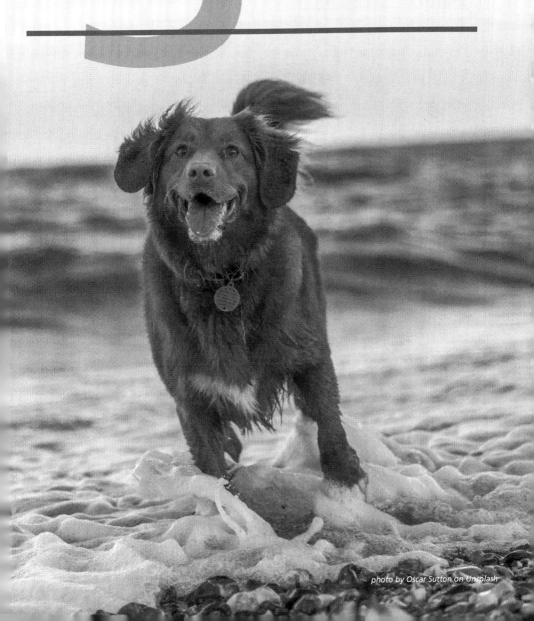

3 part three

Make an Excellent Diet Even Better

part three

chapter 10

Can We Make Even Better Choices about the Way We Feed?

Throughout these pages we've explored how you can feed your dog or cat based on the same principles you rely on when you choose a healthy diet for yourself, by eating a wide variety of fresh, whole foods—and why that's an excellent choice for health, happiness, and longevity. We've seen how those principles can benefit your dog or cat, with reduced risk of nutritional deficiencies, chronic illness, and premature aging, and improvement in overall vitality and longevity.

We've also explored how our understanding of nutrition and its relationship to health is always evolving. One of the most significant developments in recent years is the recognition that, for humans, reducing consumption of animal products can have a dramatic impact on health. As far back as 2004, biochemist T. Colin Campbell released results of his pioneering research in his book *The China Study: The Most Comprehensive Study of Nutrition Ever Conducted.* His findings revolutionized our understanding of the impact of eating animal products of all kinds—meat, dairy, and eggs—on health. Dr. Campbell found that the chances of developing heart disease, cancer, diabetes, autoimmune disease, kidney disease, and even dementia are far lower among people who consume few or no animal products compared to those who do.

Since then, our understanding of this correlation has snowballed, and become a key consideration in any discussion of healthy food choices. Today, medical doctors frequently prescribe a vegan diet, or one that minimizes animal products, for prevention of these devastating illnesses—and even as a way to reverse them.

It makes sense, then, to consider whether a vegan diet might offer similar benefits for our dogs and cats. Might they also experience better health outcomes if we eliminate or reduce the animal products they eat? Is it safe for them? If so, how do we choose vegan foods that are right for them? Will they like it? Those are critical questions, and they demand thoughtful answers.

But maybe your first question is…why? Everyone knows dogs and cats eat meat, right? All those ads we see promoting packaged foods are falling over themselves in an effort to show us their products are loaded with meat—after all, that's what caregivers want to feed, isn't it? So why should we consider what some might call a "radical" shift in the way we feed our canine and feline friends?

Most people who choose to reduce their own consumption of animal-derived foods do so for one or more of three reasons: environmental concerns, compassion for animals used for food, and, yes, for the health benefits. Let's explore how those issues apply to our nonhuman friends.

Environmental Impact

The most efficient way to use our planet's resources for food is to raise plants and eat them. When instead we raise plants to feed the animals that we in turn raise to feed ourselves, we use between ten and twenty times more land, water, fuel, and fertilizer than if we simply get our nutrients directly from the plants. Our reliance on meat, dairy, eggs, and fish is rapidly depleting our resources; contaminating our land, rivers, and groundwater; and decimating ocean populations. It also contributes heavily to the production of methane and other greenhouse gases that are a major cause of climate change.

"In the United States, dogs and cats consume approximately 25% of all the animal products used for food."

No doubt you're familiar with those concerns. What's less

well known is that our dogs and cats play an inordinately large role in all of that, because in the United States they consume approximately 25% of all the animal products used for food. How can that be? Even though our nonhuman companions are smaller than we are, and they consume a smaller volume of food, their diets tend to include a far higher proportion of animal products than ours.

If we're all taking steps to reduce our environmental footprint, it makes sense to consider whether our dogs and cats can participate by reducing their consumption of animal-derived ingredients.

Impact on Other Species

It's no secret that animals used for food are generally treated as commodities, with minimal regard for their comfort or happiness. In the United States, nearly 99% of them are raised on factory farms, created to house as many animals as possible in as small a space as possible to optimize profitability. Most of us would find it painful to witness the conditions endured by those who must spend their lives in such a facility; few people would willingly participate in the slaughter. But both of those are realities of our food supply system.

Cows, pigs, chickens, goats, and the many other species used for food are not very different from our dogs and cats in their ability to feel joy and fear, to play when circumstances allow, and form friendships with others. When a calf is taken from his mother within 24 hours of birth, as is standard practice on a dairy farm, both cry out as any mother and child would if separated too early. But that, too, is a reality of our food system, because the only way you and I can buy milk and cheese at the grocery store is to make sure that mother's milk is reserved for us—not given to her calf.

If we believe eating animal products is necessary for health—for humans, canines, or felines—then we find ways to justify treating other species this way...or we choose not to give it too much thought.

But what if eating meat isn't necessary? What if our dogs and cats could thrive on a plant-based diet, just as you and I can? Would it be worthwhile to give it a try if it could reduce the suffering of other species just a little?

Toxicity in Animal-Derived Foods

If you've been feeding a meat-based diet, no doubt you do so because you believe it's the healthiest choice. Your intentions are the best, but what you're actually feeding may be very different from what you expect.

We live in a toxic world, where industrial chemicals and other contaminants are everywhere—in our soil, in the air we breathe, and in the water we drink. As you might imagine, those contaminants are also in the plants that grow in that soil and in the animals who eat those plants. It's not just a problem in urban areas, or near industrial facilities. These dangerous chemicals are so ubiquitous they've even been found in our wildlands and in wildlife all around the globe.

"Due to the process of bioaccumulation, the higher up the food chain we eat, the more PFAS and other harmful chemicals we're likely to ingest."

For example, perfluoroalkyl and polyfluoroalkyl substances, or PFAS, are chemicals widely used in consumer goods such as cookware and packaging to make them nonstick, in cosmetics to make them waterproof, in carpeting and clothing to make them resistant to stains, and as a fire retardant. They're known to cause cancer; birth defects; heart disease; and damage to the liver, thyroid, and immune system. And they're everywhere, on every continent, including in the Arctic glaciers.

It's pretty clear that you and your dog or cat are unlikely to be able to avoid exposure to PFAS entirely. But you can reduce exposure dramatically by being careful about the foods you choose. Due to the process of bioaccumulation, the higher up the food chain we eat, the more PFAS and other harmful chemicals we're likely to ingest. Think about it: If PFAS are in the water, animals who drink that water—or, in the case of fish, live in it—ingest those chemicals with every sip. Plants absorb the chemicals in the soil and water, too. But the animals who eat those plants day after day build up a greater toxic load in their bodies over time. Take it one step further—if your dog or cat eats the animals who have been accumulating toxins in their flesh every day for months and years, and continues to eat that toxic flesh every day for months or years, your beloved friend will consume a frightening amount of dangerous chemicals that accumulate throughout his lifetime. It's hard to imagine his health would not be compromised.

In January 2023, the Environmental Working Group released a study that evaluated levels of PFAS in freshwater fish throughout the United States. They found contamination in all but two of the five hundred samples they tested. What's even more disturbing is that the level of contamination was so high that if your dog or cat was to eat a single serving of that fish, he would ingest as much PFAS as he would if he drank the contaminated water that fish came from every day for a month. That's the power of bio-accumulation.

This is just one example of how changing the way we think about healthy food for our animal friends can make an enormous difference in their vitality and longevity—and also in the health of our planet and the well-being of other animal species. In the coming chapters we'll take a look at how and why a vegan diet can be a safe choice for your dog or cat, as well as some real-life outcomes in animals who made the switch.

I think you'll be intrigued.

chapter 11

Can Dogs and Cats Go Vegan?

Dogs are descended from wolves. Contrary to popular belief, cats are not descended from lions or tigers, but from the African wildcat, a type of feline still alive and well in Africa and Asia. Our domestic cats do, however, share about 96.4% of the DNA of modern tigers and lions. We might say they're distant cousins, if not direct descendants.

In any case, our companions are closely related to those wild predators who dine primarily on other animals. Surely, it would seem, they can't possibly thrive on a plant-based diet. Or can they?

Is It "Natural"?

Much of the uncertainty around feeding a vegan diet to dogs and cats is due to concern that it's not "natural." There's an assumption that they need to be on an "ancestral diet," a term coined to refer to a diet heavily reliant on meat.

The fact is we've been sharing our homes with canines and felines for tens of thousands of years. As a result, their dietary needs have changed. Clearly that Dachshund curled up on the sofa is not a wolf, and the tabby cat purring on your lap is not a tiger; she's not even an African Wildcat.

Consider our dogs, who are genetically far removed from their wild counterparts due to centuries of selective breeding and adaptation. A wolf does rely on other animals as his primary food source. But as an omnivore—an animal who eats both plants and other animals—he also routinely consumes grasses, acorns, berries and other fruits, and the stomach contents of his plant-eating prey.

Dogs are even better suited to eating plants, including the grains and other higher-carbohydrate foods they've been sharing with us. Over millennia of living alongside humans, the digestive system of the modern dog changed, as ours did. When we began to cultivate the land and rely more on a grain-based diet, so did our canine companions, and their digestive systems evolved accordingly. One significant change was an increase in their ability to digest starches, which relies in part on the presence of the enzyme amylase, produced by the pancreas. A comprehensive study of the gene profiles of wolves and dogs found that, while wolves have two copies of a gene responsible for the production of amylase, domestic dogs have between four and thirty copies of the same gene. That means your dog is far better equipped than his wild cousins are to digest a plant-based diet—up to fifteen times better.

> "While wolves have two copies of a gene responsible for the production of amylase, dogs have between four and thirty copies of the same gene."

The wild ancestors of cats are, of course, true carnivores—and so are our domestic cats. However, like dogs, our cats have also evolved a greater ability to metabolize carbohydrates. You're probably well aware of your cat's propensity to eat grass (and occasionally your favorite houseplant); you might even have discovered that he loves corn, melon, and other plants. What many don't realize is that commercial cat foods are typically 20% to 40% carbohydrates, and include ingredients like grains, potatoes, and legumes. Still, cats lack the ability to produce some essential nutrients, such as taurine and arachidonic acid, that are not widely available in plant foods. Even so, if we assess a cat's needs in terms of nutrients rather than ingredients, we can provide a nutritionally sound diet using plant-based foods with the addition of the necessary supplements. There's an easy way to do that, as we'll see on page 91, "Feeding a Vegan Cat."

Domestication has also changed the animals you might feed to your dog or cat, so the meat she eats is substantially different from the wild game eaten by her wild relatives. A wolf or tiger might prey on a water buffalo, antelope, quail, beaver, or wild hare, all decidedly different from the cows, chickens, and sheep in today's dog and cat foods. The animals who provide the meat in today's diets labeled as "ancestral" or "species appropriate" are often dosed heavily with antibiotics; they eat grains that are genetically modified and treated with chemical pesticides and fertilizers, and their bodies are laced with stress hormones due to the lifelong stresses inherent in modern feed and slaughter operations—all of which are present in the meat your companion eats. It's hardly the same as a freshly killed wild jackrabbit, and it certainly should not be considered part of a "natural" diet.

Feeding a Vegan Dog

Because your dog is an omnivore, his body can adapt quite easily to a vegan diet. In fact, many dogs seem to blossom when they make the switch. Like anyone else, he has a long list of nutritional needs that must be met if he's to stay healthy, but the Fresh & Flexible meal plan is designed to provide for those needs. If you feed a good selection of fresh, whole foods, organic if possible, with plenty of variety—different foods and nutrition boosters in the bowl every day or every few days—your dog will have the best opportunity to get everything he needs to thrive. (For details regarding what and how to feed, see Chapter 7, "The Fresh & Flexible Meal Plan," beginning on page 43.) Simply use plant ingredients for the protein component of his meals, and avoid foods and supplements that come from animals.

"Domestication has also changed the animals you might feed to your dog or cat, so the meat she eats is substantially different from the wild game eaten by her wild relatives."

In general, dogs don't require supplementation, with one exception: Some vegan dogs require taurine, an amino acid that is not present in plants. The vast majority of dogs are able to manufacture their own taurine from cysteine, methionine, and other components that are readily available in a plant-based diet. However, certain breeds, including Golden and Labrador Retrievers, Cocker Spaniels, and some large breed dogs, have a reduced

VEGEDOG™ FEEDING GUIDE	
Dog's Weight	Daily Serving
5 lbs (2.3 kg)	½ tsp (2 g)
10 lbs (4.5 kg)	⅔ tsp (2.7 g)
15 lbs (6.8 kg)	1 tsp (4 g)
20 lbs (9.1 kg)	1⅓ tsp (5.5 g)
30 lbs (13.6 kg)	1⅔ tsp (7 g)
40 lbs (18.1 kg)	2 tsp (9 g)
50 lbs (22.7 kg)	2½ tsp (11.5 g)
60 lbs (27.2 kg)	1 tbsp (13.5 g)
80 lbs (36.3 kg)	1¼ tbsp (16.5 g)
Add an additional ⅓ tsp (1.5 g) Vegedog for every 10 lbs (4.5 kg) of bodyweight over 80 lbs	
Adapted from Compassion Circle, Inc.	

ability to do so. If your dog appears to be one of these, or if you don't know your dog's heritage, adding a taurine supplement to his vegan diet is an easy safety measure.

Vitamin B_{12} is another important nutrient that is not widely available in plant foods. Most dogs make it themselves, but it's also a good idea to augment a vegan diet with foods that supply an added boost. Spirulina and nutritional yeast are included among the recommended nutrition boosters in the Fresh & Flexible plan (see the chart on pages 48-49), and both are good sources of vitamin B_{12}. Feed one or the other on a regular basis; alternatively, you can give a weekly B_{12} supplement or add a vitamin-mineral supplement as indicated in the Fresh & Flexible guidelines on pages 56-57. Avoid any made with xylitol, a common sweetener that is highly toxic to dogs and cats.

Or, if you'd like to be extra cautious, you can add Vegedog, a supplement made for vegan dogs by the company called Compassion Circle, Inc. It provides ingredients that are less readily available on a plant-based diet, including some that your dog's body can make on its own, or that are present in nutrition boosters. Since the vast majority of dogs can get everything they need on the Fresh & Flexible meal plan without Vegedog, it's offered as an optional addition to his meals. If you'd like to order it you can do so at CompassionCircle.com. Follow the guidelines in the "Vegedog Feeding Guide" table above.

Feeding a Vegan Cat

Because cats are true carnivores, adapting to a vegan diet can be a bit more complicated for them. There are a few nutrients that are present only in foods derived from animals and that, unlike dogs, cats are unable to make in their own bodies. For that reason it is considered essential that vegan cats receive Vegecat, the supplement designed just for them by Compassion Circle, Inc., at CompassionCircle.com. Follow the guidelines in the "Vegecat Feeding Guide" table below.

Some cats switch easily to plant-based meals, while others take longer to adjust and need more support. A few don't seem suited to it. It's up to you to observe what your cat tells you, and do what is best for him. You have plenty of resources in this book to help you introduce a vegan diet safely. A successful transition may provide a boon to your friend's health now and in the years to come. But if you find he doesn't adapt well, or is unwilling to make the adjustment, don't force it on him. You may still get some of the benefits by reducing the proportion of meat in his meals in favor of healthier plant-derived high-protein foods.

VEGECAT™ FEEDING GUIDE	
Cat's Weight	**Daily Serving**
5 lbs (2.3 kg)	⅜ tsp (1.6 g)
10 lbs (4.5 kg)	⅔ tsp (2.7 g)
15 lbs (6.8 kg)	⅚ tsp (3.6)
20 lbs (9.1 kg)	1¹⁄₁₆ tsp (4.4g)
Adapted from Compassion Circle, Inc.	

But Will He Like It?

I stopped eating meat more than thirty years ago and have been vegan for about twenty-five years. My dogs and cats have joined me on that journey, and all of them have enjoyed their meals along with the noticeable health benefits. I'm pretty sure I've never seen anyone appreciate any treat more than Tila Marie loved a raw stalk of broccoli. The look of joy on her face as she munched on those florets was something I'll never forget. Tino Val-

"Caregivers are often amazed to see how much their companions enjoy vegetables and fruits, or other foods not typically considered 'dog food' or 'cat food.'"

entino was a wise ten years old when he adopted me, and I'm quite certain he had never seen a vegan meal in his life until then. Still, like most Boxers, he was unequivocally enthusiastic about everything and anything I put in his bowl, starting with his very first dinner with me. His only complaint—ever—was that there wasn't more of it. And here's one that might surprise you: Dogs love sauerkraut. I'm not kidding. Most cats do, too. I guess they just know what good food is.

By and large, all animals are drawn to good, healthy food, so you can expect to make the switch to fresh, healthy—even vegan—food with little or no resistance. Caregivers are often amazed to see how much their companions enjoy vegetables and fruits, or other foods not typically considered "dog food" or "cat food." That's why the transition to a Fresh & Flexible diet, and even a vegan Fresh & Flexible plan, is often seamless and welcomed by the recipient.

Of course, there are exceptions. Dogs, by and large, are easy to please. Most are happy to eat whatever is for dinner. Still, some are hesitant when offered a food that's unfamiliar. With a little coaxing and some extra enthusiasm from their humans, it's usually not difficult to persuade them to give it a try.

But let's face it: Cats can be a bit fussy. Well…some are a lot fussy. Many take readily to their new vegan food; I've even seen one pass up a plate of commercial, meat-based cat food for a home-prepared tofu dinner. (It's true—and there's a video to prove it.) Others have more trouble, and some decline to give up their carnivorous ways.

If your dog or cat is reluctant to eat his vegan meals, here are a few tricks that might coax him along:

- **Introduce the new food gradually.** Since the biggest change will be in the protein portion of his meal, try introducing a small amount of tofu, beans, or other vegan option along with his usual portion of meat.

Gradually decrease the amount of meat in favor of increasing portions of your vegan protein sources. Chances are that in time he'll be enjoying his meals without realizing the meat is gone.

- **Be sure to try different vegan foods to replace the meat in his meals.** Like the rest of us, your companion prefers some foods over others. Take time letting him explore different flavors and textures, and find out which ones he enjoys the most.

- **Add something tasty on top of his meal.** Most dogs and cats love fatty foods and oil, so a drizzle of his olive, coconut, or other oil on top of his meal might be more enticing than mixing it in. Other tasty toppings include spirulina, nutritional yeast, tomato sauce, soy or other nondairy milk, vegetable broth, a few dabs of peanut butter or peanut butter gravy (see page 69), or a sprinkle of vegan parmesan.

- **Invite him to eat what you're eating.** I'd be surprised if your friend wasn't generally interested in whatever it is that you're eating, and you can use that to your advantage. Before you serve his meal, sit down and start eating it as if it's your dinner. Don't hide the fact that you love every bite—the more dramatic you are the more he'll want some, too. Offer a small taste and then eat some more yourself, with plenty of oohs and ahhs over how delicious it is. When he can barely keep his nose out of your dish, go ahead and let him enjoy his yummy dinner.

You'll find more suggestions under "If Your Friend Has Discriminating Tastes" on pages 68-70 in Chapter 8.

Making the Switch

To make the switch to meatless fare for your friend, simply choose plant-based sources for the protein component of his meals. Beans, nuts, seeds, tofu, tempeh, and seitan are all good choices. The suggestions under "Protein" on pages 46-51 in Chapter 7 will give you plenty of ideas for different higher-protein foods to try. Keep in mind, though, that nearly all plants contain some protein, and many leafy green vegetables contain a higher percentage of protein than some types of animal flesh. That's one more reason why your friend can easily get all the protein she needs on a vegan diet.

Here are a few additional guidelines you may find helpful:

- Since plants tend to have more fiber than meat, dairy, or eggs, the proportions of protein-rich ingredients you put in the bowl may need to be a little higher.

- Cook grains and beans until soft, and purée the larger, firmer varieties of beans. (See "Dried beans and other legumes…" page 60 in Chapter 7 for tips on how to cook the tastiest, most digestible beans.)

- If you need to rely on a commercial dog food, or just have one on hand for occasional use, there are vegetarian and vegan varieties available. However, the same concerns about processing, preservatives, chemical additives, poor quality ingredients, and lack of variety apply, just as they do with meat-based formulas. Be sure to read the list of ingredients carefully, and make sure there are no by-products or additives that might be harmful.

- Remember to include the most important ingredient in any healthy diet: Variety, variety, variety. That way you'll be sure your friend gets the balance of amino acids he needs. Give him lentils on Tuesday, black beans on the weekend, tofu on Sunday morning.

Once your companion starts his new diet, watch for changes—for better or worse—in his health or behavior. A brittle coat, low energy, or weak muscles may be a sign he's not getting enough protein. Review the guidelines under "Find the Right Balance" starting on page 63 in Chapter 8, and adjust his meals accordingly.

On the other hand, you may find that his coat becomes softer and shinier, his energy and mood are more balanced, he's less afraid of those thunderstorms, his breath is fresh, and that nasty build-up on his teeth seems to be going away. If that's the case—celebrate and carry on!

chapter 12

The Healing Power of Good Food

I t's well known that in humans, a vegan diet can reduce the risk of cancer, as well as diabetes, liver and kidney disease, gastrointestinal disturbances, arthritis, and obesity—all conditions that affect our dogs and cats. Whether this is due to lower levels of toxicity, higher levels of antioxidants and phytonutrients, improved gut microbiome, or a direct result of eliminating animal proteins, it's impossible to say. Sadly, there is little research available to tell us whether eliminating animal products from our companions' diets will provide similar benefits. It's reasonable to expect it will.

That's certainly consistent with changes I see when clients transition their animals to a vegan diet. Here are a few examples:

- **Obesity.** Grace was a decidedly overweight pup when rescued from a shelter in New Mexico, U.S., but easily lost 16 pounds within the first year on her vegan diet. The reduced fat and calories and ample portions of fruits and vegetables allowed her to trim down without ever lacking in nutrition or feeling deprived.

- **Gastrointestinal (GI) disturbance.** I often see digestive problems resolve quickly with no treatment other than a change to a vegan diet, usually without an extended transition period. Atticus' case was particularly dramatic. This sweet and mellow Cane Corso had ongoing upper and lower GI troubles throughout his first 6½ years. He typically moved his bowels four times a day, and most stools were liquid. He often refused to eat, and had frequent bouts of vomiting. On two occasions those were so severe they required a trip to the emergency room. Despite extensive testing and repeated veterinary exams, no one was ever able to identify any illness, obstruction, or cause for Atty's distress. It was only when he was switched to a vegan diet that he was finally able to utilize his food as most dogs do—his appetite returned with gusto, his bowel movements became normal, and the vomiting ended.

- **Food sensitivity.** Patches was a long-haired calico cat who had suffered from food sensitivities most of her life. Soon after eating, she'd dash around her apartment, stopping only to frantically lick her coat or scratch. Initially, changing to a different commercial food solved the problem, but each time, within a few months, symptoms reappeared. By the time she was nine years old, Patches was reactive to every meat-based commercial or home-prepared food her caregiver offered. When she was switched to a vegan diet, the itching stopped, never to return.

- **Reduced mobility.** At age 11½, Ocean was exhibiting a decline in mobility, as is common among senior dogs. He had difficulty getting up, and walking was painful. X-rays indicated he had advanced arthritis in his hips and spine. Within two months on a vegan diet, Ocean's mobility and energy level improved, and he and his dad were able to enjoy their walks along the coast at Figueira da Foz, Portugal.

- **Seizure disorder.** Mira, a 7-year-old Border Collie cross, was having multiple seizures each day, while suffering severe side effects of potassium bromide and phenobarbital, drugs intended to treat her disorder. She was put on a vegan diet and treated with homeopathy. Within weeks she was free of seizures, and was soon able to discontinue the pharmaceutical medications. About a year later, her guardian suffered a serious accident and was hospitalized. The woman who took over Mira's care was unable to provide a vegan diet, and Mira's seizures returned. She was put back on the pharmaceuticals, but the seizures persisted and continued to get more severe. Mira passed away a few months later.

- **Age-related degenerative changes.** At 14, Dakota, a Chow cross, had pain and muscle soreness in her lower back. Her hind legs had become weak, and she had trouble controlling her movement. Climbing the stairs was difficult for her, and left her panting and distressed. Her energy was low, and her once-luxurious coat had become rough and dull. Things took an even darker turn when Dakota's lab results came back with signs of early kidney disease. After two weeks on a vegan diet, Dakota's mobility had improved; she had less lower-back pain and a softer coat. After three weeks she was stronger, more playful, with still less discomfort, and was climbing stairs more easily and with no panting. After six months, her kidney function had normalized. Her guardian reported that a friend they hadn't seen in some time saw Dakota playing and asked if this was a new puppy—and was amazed to learn that the "puppy" was a revitalized Dakota.

When you introduce the Fresh & Flexible meal plan to your cat or dog, you make the choice for healthier food and all the benefits it can bring. If you take it one step further and make her meals vegan, you just might make an outstanding diet even better.

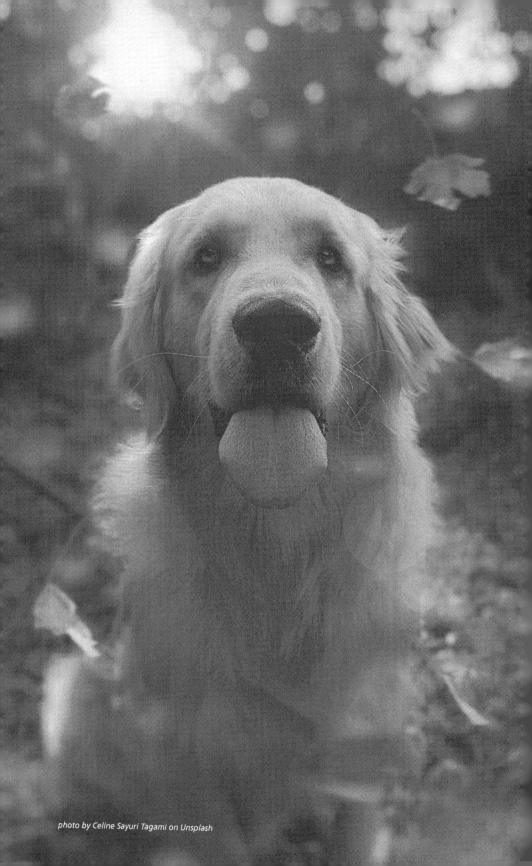

Epilog

An Unexpected Benefit

Making good choices about the food we eat and feed to our families is the first step in keeping us healthy. But food is not just about nourishing our bodies. It brings us together to share a common bond, a way to celebrate tradition and ritual. It's one of the ways we care for each other, and nurture one another emotionally and spiritually. It's about connection...friendship...family...love. We choose the foods we prepare for those we love based on what will sustain them physically, but also to bring them pleasure, and to share the foods our parents gave us when they knew we needed to feel loved.

Most of us, if we were fortunate enough to be raised by people who were kind to us, can recall the taste and smell of something nourishing and nurturing, given to us with love and tenderness. Years later...decades, even... we return to those familiar dishes when we need a little extra comfort.

We build our cultural and, often, spiritual traditions around food. When I was growing up, my mother made homemade bread every year on Christmas Eve, and used the same dough to make pizza for our dinner. At Easter, we spent all day Saturday building huge trays of calzone, in a sweet crust layered with ricotta and eggs and ham, then enjoyed it Sunday morning along with a lamb-shaped cake covered in coconut. Holidays at my grandmother's home were veritable feasts, with an endless array of heaping platters spread across her dining table and the buffet against the wall.

But some of my favorite food memories were the simplest...like the guilty pleasure of having buttered noodles for dinner when it was just my mom and me, with no one to criticize the lack of a vegetable. When I was sick, she'd make me a cup of steaming hot lemon and honey. If I tried to make it for myself, I could never get it quite as sweet as she did, no matter how much honey I added.

Food is an expression of love. We feel it when someone makes a favorite dish for us. Maybe we feel it even more when we tenderly prepare a meal for someone we treasure, then see the pleasure it brings. Best of all is when we sit down to share a special meal together with a cherished friend or family member.

When you feed your dog or cat the Fresh & Flexible way, you invite him or her into your circle of family and friendship…your traditions…in a way nothing else does. You open up a whole new way to be present with him emotionally, attentively. When you walk through the aisles of your grocery store, you scan the shelves thinking about what he'd enjoy…which foods will help him stay healthy, and how you'll prepare them just the way he likes them. When you open the refrigerator to decide what's for dinner, you look for something he hasn't had in a while, so you can put something different in his bowl. Chances are he'll be close by, watching patiently, eager to see what you come up with. As you put on a pot to simmer or heat up a pan, you'll be thinking about how you'll put flavors together to bring him pleasure, all the while knowing you're using your own hands, your own energy, and your knowledge to create a meal that will help him stay healthy and also delight him. Soon you'll watch him put his nose in his bowl and eat that meal with gusto…then look up at you, tail swishing, with a smile of appreciation on that gorgeous face of his. And you'll know…you did that. You put your intellect and your heart, your intention and your energy to the task of giving him health and happiness, with food…one of the most caring, intimate gifts you can give.

I am without a dog or cat in my family at the moment. My Tino left this world a few months ago. But as I type these words, my heart is filled with the love I felt, and still feel, every day as I made those meals for him, and watched the complete and utter enjoyment he took from each and every one. I know he sensed the love and care that went into them. It is one of the things I miss most about having someone like him in my life.

There are a lot of reasons to feed the Fresh & Flexible way. It's hard to think of a reason more important than keeping your precious dog or cat as healthy as she can be. But the way it will change your relationship with her is an unexpected gift that will benefit both of you. When you free yourself to choose the foods you know are best for her, and select what goes into her bowl each day depending on what you know she needs and what she loves, then prepare it with love and see her delight in it all…you'll find that it changes things in a subtle but profound way: It deepens your connection. It strengthens your bond.

The Fresh & Flexible meal plan is a way to brush away one more boundary between ourselves and our dogs and cats...and perhaps other species as well. It reminds us that we're more alike than we are different. As we let go of the notion that "dog food" and "cat food" are different from human food, we discover that we can sit together with them at the same table—figuratively if not literally—and share one more part of our lives in a way we never did before. And we do it through food, that tender, intimate way we humans have of expressing our love for one another. What could be more delicious than that.

About the Author

Jan Allegretti, D.Vet.Hom., has been a consultant and educator in holistic health care for nonhuman animals since 1988, specializing in nutrition, homeopathy, and lifestyle assessment. She is the author of *The Holistic Animal Health Series*, which includes the bestselling *The Complete Holistic Dog Book: Home Health Care for Our Canine Companions*, a comprehensive manual for health and healing through nutrition, homeopathy, herbal medicine, and a supportive home environment. She works with home caregivers, shelter and rescue organizations, and veterinary professionals throughout the United States and internationally through private consultations, workshops, and as a speaker at conferences and outreach events. Her work has been published in professional and trade publications including the *International Animal Health Journal*, the *Journal of the Academy of Veterinary Homeopathy*, and *Vegan Life Magazine*.

Jan is deeply committed to animal advocacy, writing and working to foster a better relationship between humans and other species. In 2006 and 2007 she successfully led a coalition to prevent the building of a slaughterhouse in her community; in 2007 co-founded the Mendocino County, California, animal advocacy organization CARE: Compassion for Animals, Respect for the Earth; and has been nominated for the American Red Cross (Sonoma and Mendocino Counties) Real Heroes Award in the Animal Category.

Supporting caregivers in offering healthy, home-prepared meals and, when possible, a vegan diet, to companion animals is a natural melding of Jan's work as a healer and as an advocate for animals of all species. She finds great enjoyment in empowering humans to integrate their compassion into all aspects of their relationships with other animals—and in seeing the animals they care for thrive as a result. Her commitment to enhancing awareness and relationship among all species is evident in her writing, including her book *Listen to the Silence: Lessons from Trees and Other Masters* and the extensive library of articles archived on her website, JanAllegretti.com.

Jan lives in the hills of northern California, where she shares her mountaintop home with the resident deer, ravens, coyotes, rattlesnakes, bears, jackrabbits, and countless other wise and wild ones.

Acknowledgements

This book is the fruit of more than three decades of exploration and observation, study and learning. As with any evolution, there are many who lent contributions and support, and who gave me clues, nudges, play bows, tail wags, and slow blinks along the way.

Mark Coleman is the gifted graphic designer who created these beautiful pages. He's also endlessly patient and generous. Thank you, Mark, for being on call to burn the midnight oil to flow text and meet deadlines, and for always doing it with grace. I can't imagine creating this book without you.

Jacqueline Barton is one of those rare friends who is ready to help any time in any way, sharing the love of our dogs and cats and horses, and the turkeys and the goats, and who also happens to make the best coffee. Thank you, Jackie, for reading all those pages, then reading them again, and for cheering me on when it seemed I'd never get it all done. But I think I'm most grateful that we can cry together in grief and also laugh until we cry... the best of times.

Richard and Susan Pitcairn helped spread the word about Fresh & Flexible, inviting me to introduce it to veterinarians who introduced it to clients who introduced it to...yes, their dogs and cats. Ripples in the pond, indeed. That led to lots more enthusiasm, and lots of healthier dogs and cats. When Susan realized it needed a name, she helped christen it as Fresh & Flexible. My deep gratitude to you both.

When Lisa Melling first heard what Fresh & Flexible was all about, she was the greatest of skeptics. She asked the best and toughest questions, poked at it from every angle, then came away as one of its greatest champions. She's supported it ever since, sharing it with other veterinarians and with her clients who shared it with...well, you know. Thank you, Lisa, for your beautiful, infectious enthusiasm. You always make me smile.

I'm deeply grateful to Todd Cooney and the many veterinarians who have been open minded enough to consider this approach, and willing to step outside the box to share it with their clients. Thank you for playing a key role in opening this new avenue to good health.

Jenny Burnstad has made so many things much, much easier. Through her work and the support of the Cloud Forest Institute, she brought love and light and clarity to countless administrative details. Thank you, Jen.

The support of the Fred and Jean Allegretti Foundation has made it possible to do so much more—not only with this book, but also my advocacy work and that of so many other individuals and organizations. Their generosity leaves a legacy that has and will continue to save and brighten many lives.

There's one person who has been there almost longer than I can remember, and whose longevity is matched only by his constancy...my rock. I would have given up long ago if not for you.

Of course, Fresh & Flexible would never have happened without the many dogs and cats who ate all the good food. They were clear about what they loved, and when they were feeling fussy they helped me figure out how to make it more delicious. Most of all they showed me how it helped them become healthier, happier, and more radiant. I'm grateful to countless client pups and kitties and their humans who did the meal prep and relayed feedback. And of course, it all started, and continues to evolve, with my precious family members who took me on the journey and shared meals right here in our kitchen...Patches, Mazie the Amazing Kitty, Ginger, Tashina, Savannah, Tila Marie, Tiffany, and Valentino "Tino" Angelino. I will always treasure every minute of every meal we shared.

Index

Made in the USA
Middletown, DE
30 August 2024

60068375R00073